The
Narcissist
in Your Life

T0384201

The Narcissist
in Your Life

Recognizing the Patterns
and Learning to Break Free

JULIE L. HALL

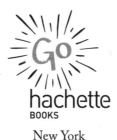

hachette
BOOKS

New York

Copyright © 2019 by Julie L. Hall
Cover design by Kerry Rubenstein
Cover photograph copyright © ArtMari/Shutterstock
Cover copyright © 2019 Hachette Book Group, Inc.

Hachette Go, an imprint of Hachette Books
Hachette Book Group
1290 Avenue of the Americas
New York, NY 10104
HachetteGo.com
Facebook.com/HachetteGo
Instagram.com/HachetteGo

Previously published by Da Capo Lifelong edition 2019
First Hachette Go edition 2021

Hachette Books is a division of Hachette Book Group, Inc. The Hachette Go and Hachette Books name and logos are trademarks of Hachette Book Group, Inc.

The Hachette Speakers Bureau provides a wide range of authors for speaking events. To find out more, go to www.hachettespeakersbureau.com or call (866) 376-6591.

The publisher is not responsible for websites (or their content) that are not owned by the publisher.

Print book interior design by Linda Mark.

Library of Congress Cataloging-in-Publication Data has been applied for.
ISBNs: 978-0-7382-8577-1 (trade paperback), 978-0-7382-8578-8 (ebook)

LSC-C

Printing 8, 2024

For my mother and father, who brought me into
this life and shaped me, for better and worse.
I thank you for the good, forgive you for the hurt,
and hope for healing and peace for us all
in this life and whatever comes next.

Contents

Acknowledgments

FOREMOST, DEEP GRATITUDE TO MY FAMILY, SARAH AND LUCY, FOR steadfastly supporting me through my seemingly endless questions, ramblings, rants, and tears while writing the contents of this book. You listened and loved, and when you couldn't listen anymore you pretended.

A special thank-you to the survivors who entrusted me with their stories. You matter, and you always did.

Sharyn Wolf, you went above and beyond to help a girl you barely knew when she was down. You righteously walk the talk, and this red-haired primate bows before you in gratitude. To my agent and honorary godmother Joelle Delbourgo: Thank you for changing your mind. To my soul sister editor Renée Sedliar, with whom I finally get the last word: You—the best. And thank you to the rest of the team at Da Capo Lifelong.

Many thanks to Elinor Greenberg, Margalis Fjelstad, Karyl McBride, Regina Collins, Fiona Steele, Julie Tenenberg, Sharone Weltfreid, Barbara Mills, and Melissa McRitchie.

To my sister warrior Aleta McClelland: Your heart will never be contained. To my sister warrior Colleen Byrum: You are a force of nature.

An affectionate thanks to my bro Don Huddleston.

Abiding gratitude to Lucia Vracin, healer and friend.

Thank you to Barrie Hillman, headmaster at West Sound Academy, whose generosity helped my family steady the ship in turbulent times.

And to my sisters Adrienne Fuson and Erica Fuson: You are my cherished consolation-prize phoenixes rising!

Foreword

A JOURNALIST, SURVIVOR, AND NARCISSISTIC ABUSE TRAUMA CONSULTANT, Julie L. Hall has firsthand experience with the effects of narcissistic abuse, and she has done her homework to understand the patterns that appear in narcissist-dominated families.

Hall's *The Narcissist in Your Life* describes, in depth, the effects that the narcissistic behavior of a family member—parent, spouse, or child—can have on everyone else in the family. It describes different types of narcissistic behavior and how each can lead to abuse of boundaries, twisting of facts, distortions in perceptions, attacks on self-identity, confused understanding of reality, and even long-term physical health problems.

Hall clearly illustrates the techniques that narcissists use to get what they want from others without taking responsibility for their behaviors—including isolation, destabilizing reality, thought control, gaslighting, and even terror. In addition, she covers the typical reactions that family members have to the narcissist's manipulations, and the long-term effects that these patterns can have on their health, emotional well-being, and even life choices. There is a wealth of information here. The lists and examples of narcissistic behaviors and their impact on family members, outlines of family rules and roles, and personal interviews are especially helpful in bringing a deeper understanding of the depth and breadth of narcissistic exploitation and manipulation. And the strategies for family members are practical and compassionate.

As the author of *Stop Caretaking the Borderline or Narcissist* and an upcoming book on creating resiliency in children with a borderline or narcissist parent, I know how valuable this information is. Hall offers a very realistic look at NPD and how survivors need to stay aware and prepared for future infringements and manipulations from the narcissist. She will give you hope and insight into how to help yourself and your kids heal.

If you're someone who has grown up with a narcissistic or self-involved parent . . .

If you're someone who has married a charismatic but domineering and demanding person . . .

If you're someone who is struggling to figure out why your partner, who used to tell you that you were so special, now can find nothing about you that is pleasing or positive . . .

If you're someone who wants desperately to understand how your loved one can be so mean, arrogant, berating, bullying, and selfish when you work so hard to be caring, thoughtful, and kind . . .

Then this book is for you.

Margalis Fjelstad, PhD, LMFT
Therapist, Educator, International Speaker
Author of *Stop Caretaking the Borderline or Narcissist*
Fort Collins, Colorado

Introduction

WELCOME. AS SOMEONE WITH A NARCISSISTIC PARENT, PARTNER, OR other important person in your life, you followed a confusing and painful road to get here. It is not a club any of us wants to join, and yet there is hope and wisdom to be found. This book won't erase your pain or solve your problems. But if you are ready, it will help you understand what you've been through, clarify your feelings, and help you move forward with healing.

Thanks to the Internet and social media, today's rapid-fire sharing of our individual and collective experience is unprecedented. We talk a lot about a lot of things, but lately it seems the subject of narcissism pops up everywhere. Public discourse about narcissism seems to have reached an all-time high, crashing across our mass consciousness like a tsunami. With an estimated 6.2 percent of people[1] impaired with narcissistic personality disorder (NPD) and an even greater number with pathological levels of narcissistic traits, most of us are touched in some way by this mental condition, whether in or outside our families. Yet, despite its notoriety, narcissism remains insidiously hidden and misunderstood while at once intensely traumatic to be around.

A defining characteristic of NPD is exploitative and abusive behavior, which is often shuttered from outside view. Narcissistic abuse rears its ugly head in our institutions, but its roots are domestic, making it a family scourge that traumatizes children, partners, and other relatives on an erosive daily basis and often persists across generations.

Those who haven't experienced narcissistic abuse firsthand find it un-imaginable and typically diminish or altogether dismiss it. This is because the narcissist operates outside normative moral boundaries, with dysfunctional empathy and grandiose self-importance masking underlying shame that s/he himself is often blind to. Even many mental health practitioners do not understand narcissism and its devastating impact.

Survivors of narcissistic trauma feel alone in their experience, but the reality is that it manifests in remarkably similar ways from one relation-ship to the next, one family to the next. This is because people with the disorder exhibit consistent patterns of thinking and behaving that create a commonality among those who are treated to their outsize demands and manipulations. If there is a saving grace for narcissistic abuse survivors, it is this common ground: Survivors in a sense are all part of one big unhappy family, and finding that commonality can offer vital validation and insight along the healing path.

As young people we all go through narcissistic developmental phases, and as adults we have narcissistic traits that help us survive and self-advocate in a vast, often battering world. The kind of narcissism I examine in this book is neither normal "healthy" narcissism nor run-of-the-mill self-centeredness. The focus of this book is narcissistic personality disorder, a pathologically crippling mental impairment, and its traumatic effect on those treated to its distortions and abuses.

This book is meant to provide a road map for survivors of narcissistic abuse looking for answers and strategies for coping. Here you will find de-tailed explanations of the disorder, including causes and traits. We'll analyze narcissistic behaviors in relationships and examine the roles that play out in families dominated by one or more narcissists. We'll identify patterns of narcissistic abuse and neglect and their traumatizing effects and look at numerous real-life examples from survivors and interviews with clinicians. Along the way, we'll lay out strategies you can use to help yourself and those you love heal and overcome trauma.

The purpose of this book is not to demonize narcissists. They have a profound impairment that causes them suffering, and often they them-selves have been victims of abuse. It is natural to sympathize with the pain that drives them to such lengths of grandiose pretense and violent defensiveness. But narcissists do terrible harm, with little to no remorse.

They are disturbed, deluded, and exploitative, particularly of family members, regardless of the emotional, psychological, and physical damage they cause.

This book is for the people narcissists have hurt: the survivors, who come in all classes, colors, creeds, sexual orientations, and gender identities. Whether you have (or had) a narcissistic parent, partner, or relative, or you love someone who does, this book is for you. If you are wondering whether someone important in your life is a narcissist and how to deal with it, this book is for you. Whether you are a scapegoat, "golden child," or unwitting enabler (we'll get to those terms in a bit), this book is for you. May it be a light of insight, support, and validation in your life. You deserve all of those things and more.

MY STORY

Over the years as an educational writer, journalist, and poet, I never imagined choosing to write about narcissism. But when I found myself working on a memoir, there was no way around taking a hard look at my own experiences growing up in a narcissistic family, experiences that caused lasting emotional and physiological damage in my life. I started writing articles and founded a blog about narcissism, *The Narcissist Family Files* (narcissist-familyfiles.com). I had already come to understand much about narcissism through my own personal pursuit of healing from my past—intensive reading, research, self-reflection, therapy, and talking with certain key people who understood. But as soon as I began exploring the subject in earnest as a journalist, I realized I had more to learn and process and a passionate drive to help others struggling with narcissism-related trauma.

This book is drawn from my personal experience, research, interviews with clinicians and survivors, consulting, and writings about narcissism—in particular the narcissistic family, where pathological narcissism is engendered and tragically perpetuated across generations. I know firsthand how deeply wounding, complex, and persistent narcissistic trauma is. I've felt trapped and sometimes broken, and I've walked down more than my fair share of blind alleys. In the process, I have also learned a lot about resiliency, empathy, and the power of hope and healing. The smallest ray of light pierces darkness and leads the way.

HOW TO USE THIS BOOK

This book is organized in six parts that can be read sequentially from start to finish or taken in pieces most immediately helpful to you. I've provided a detailed Contents so you can readily find topics you may want to read about right away, such as the narcissistic family roles, coparenting with a narcissist ex, or managing an aging narcissistic parent. You may find it useful to begin by reviewing the defined terms in the Glossary, particularly if you plan to skip around. Or you may want to start at the beginning of the book and take things chapter by chapter. Throughout you will find survivor stories, with names and identifying details changed for anonymity.

However you choose to use this book, I hope you will read its entirety. You are likely to find that topics that at first appear unrelated to you do in fact have relevance. For example, adult children of narcissists not in a relationship with a narcissistic partner will probably still benefit from reading Part 4, "Partners of Narcissists," to gain insight into an enabling parent, codependent patterns, and childhood roles. Partners of narcissists, likewise, may find it helpful to read Part 5, "Children of Narcissists," to understand past or current family dynamics and ways to help children. And even if you are familiar with the particulars of NPD, you will probably find insight in Part 2, "Narcissistic Personality Disorder," which explicates the commonly cited list of nine criteria for NPD by the American Psychiatric Association and explores other aspects of the disorder.

The bottom line is that narcissistic relationships do not happen arbitrarily. There are nearly always larger patterns at work that link how we are raised with how we live our lives and choose partners, friends, bosses, and the like in adulthood. As a survivor and writer, I believe in the power and redemption of the examined life. My goal with this book is to provide the right combination of both scope and specificity for you as reader looking to understand your experience and move forward on the vital path of recovery.

Part 1, "Reclaiming Your Rights," establishes a context for your experience with narcissistic abuse by defining human rights and how and why narcissists violate them. I hold out a hand for those stepping beyond the first defense of denial and self-blame to begin to confront the dehumanization of life with a narcissist. And I validate your need to identify the narcissist's pathology even and especially when the narcissist her-/himself will not.

Part 2, "Narcissistic Personality Disorder," looks at narcissistic personality disorder (NPD) head-on. It interprets accepted diagnostic criteria for NPD and provides multiple additional perspectives into the disorder. It identifies causes of narcissism and takes a close look at the narcissist's impaired empathy and its effect on others. It describes types of narcissists, including the closet, exhibitionist, and malignant narcissist, and it explores how and why NPD is an abusive disorder as well as patterns of narcissistic abuse. Part 2 concludes with the profound and underexamined issue of health consequences for survivors of narcissistic abuse trauma, including interviews with clinicians and a look at complex post-traumatic stress disorder (CPTSD).

Part 3, "The Narcissistic Family," dives into another fundamental but underexplored subject: the narcissistic family, including unspoken rules and roles for family members. It identifies patterns that define family life, including isolation, rage, projection, shaming, gaslighting, triangulating, smear campaigns, cognitive distortions, and tragedy. And it addresses narcissistic "love" and contempt, as well as the realities of generational narcissism and hope for overcoming it.

Partners of narcissists are the focus of Part 4, "Partners of Narcissists," which begins by analyzing narcissistic relationship patterns, from romance to devaluation to breakup, as well as how to evaluate if your partner is a narcissist. It examines codependency and trauma bonding and ways to overcome them, as well as strategies for managing a narcissistic relationship and getting out of one. Part 4 also looks at the realities of parenting with a narcissistic partner and a narcissistic ex, including ways to support your children and help them cope with dysfunctional family roles. It concludes with a look at parental alienation.

Part 5, "Children of Narcissists," takes a hard look at the experience of children in the narcissistic family, beginning with narcissistic styles of parenting, including idealizing and devaluing, parentification, neglect, engulfment, infantilization, overindulgence, and overpraising. It examines the realities of the child roles of hero, scapegoat, golden child, lost child, and mascot, as well as the impact of the roles in adulthood and ways to overcome their trappings. Part 5 also covers why and how narcissistic parents divide their kids, how to deal with a golden child sibling, and sibling relationships in adulthood.

Finally, Part 6, "Overcoming Narcissistic Abuse," focuses on overcoming narcissistic abuse trauma. It begins with strategies for processing trauma, including understanding grief and its forms, reassessing childhood stories, ending the cycle with the next generation, and finding appropriate therapeutic help. It explores ways to manage someone who has a narcissistic personality, from interpreting the narcissist's "nice" behavior, to asserting boundaries (including going no contact), to coping with the aging narcissistic parent. Part 6 presents numerous strategies for recovery and takes a close look at trusting your instincts, processing your foreshortened sense of the future, taking a self-inventory, embracing your vulnerability, and welcoming back your inner exiles. The book concludes with final lessons about societal narcissism, the role of forgiveness, and healing takeaways.

As you read, remember to be patient with yourself. Facing painful truths about your family, your relationships, and yourself is always difficult, and it takes time. You may need to reread parts or set some things aside. You are likely to find that understanding comes unevenly, with some things rushing to the surface and others remaining stubbornly out of reach. Keep at it. You are worth it.

PART 1

RECLAIMING YOUR RIGHTS

one

Understanding Your Rights

A S SOMEONE WITH A NARCISSIST IN YOUR LIFE, WHETHER AS A PARENT or other family member, partner, friend, or other important person, one thing is certain: Your fundamental human rights have been violated. Your dignity, integrity, and basic freedoms have been crossed and curtailed in countless ways. This is why you feel beaten down, trapped, confused, angry, and sick in your soul and possibly your body. And making matters far worse is the fact that the person who violated your humanity is someone close to you—someone you have cared for and thought cared for you.

NARCISSISTS VIOLATE HUMAN RIGHTS

In 1948, the United Nations set forth a Universal Declaration of Human Rights,[1] which countries around the world use to define what it means to be human and what we as a species agree deserves protection under the law. The document identifies thirty essential human rights for everyone. Let's look at a few especially pertinent ones here in relation to the narcissistic personality.

1. Equal Entitlement to Rights and Freedoms

The idea that everyone is equally entitled to the same rights and freedoms runs fundamentally counter to the narcissist's personal belief system. Contrary to the notion of equality and shared sovereignty, narcissists see themselves as superior and entitled to special privileges. For them, the world is a rigid and simplistic hierarchy of winners and losers, strong and weak, deserving and un-deserving—and democracy suffers.[2] If narcissists were to entertain the notion that life itself grants each of us equal value, their delusion of superiority would collapse and leave them with no defense against their underlying feelings of amorphousness and deficiency. They may claim to believe in equality and even decry injustice, but in their own lives they are tyrants.

2. Equal Legal Protection

Narcissists see themselves as *above the law*. As with equal rights and free-doms, the concept of equal protection under the law contradicts the nar-cissistic expectation of privileged treatment. From narcissists' perspective, laws and social structures are useful only insofar as they protect their access to special social standing and freedoms. To the extent that they believe they can get away with it, they manipulate, exploit, and violate laws and legal systems for their own ends while readily using those same institutions to constrain and punish others. No better example of this is the narcissistic spouse/parent who lies and manipulates in court to pun-ish her/his ex and control her/his children regardless of the harm it does to them.

3. Freedom from Cruel or Degrading Treatment

With infantile neediness, outsize entitlement, and dysfunctional empathy, narcissists are routinely cruel and degrading to others. They view life as a zero-sum game in which there is never enough power, self-esteem, respect, or love to go around, and others must fail for them to succeed. They do not hesitate to guilt, humiliate, or exploit others to "win," and they behave abu-sively to assert their dominance.

4. Privacy and Freedom from Personal Attack on Honor or Reputation

Narcissists have little respect for the privacy and autonomy of other people. Seeing life through their own narrowly selfish lens and lacking compassion for others' perspectives and feelings, they tend to objectify those around them rather than recognize their individual humanity. If it suits their needs, they violate boundaries and attack with distortions, innuendo, lies, and smear campaigns.

5. Free Thought

This fundamental right seems so intrinsic to being alive as to render it beyond question. But in relationship to a narcissist, thinking our own thoughts and holding our own beliefs are threats to be suppressed. Narcissists insist on agreement, and they use interrogation, bullying, guilt, and endless other tactics to get it. In their ideal universe, they would control the thoughts of everyone around them. This is because they have scripts or narratives about themselves and the people in their lives that they believe everyone should follow. The specifics of narcissists' scripts vary, but they always support inflated self-beliefs of exceptionalism and entitlement, constructions meant to allay underlying shame and self-doubt. Their scripts portray them as special—smarter, stronger, better looking, more noble, more generous, funnier, sexier, more accomplished, and the list goes on. They expect others to follow the script, upholding their need to be recognized as someone worthy of admiration and privilege. Anyone who goes off script threatens the narcissist's need to control the narrative. Such a person must be either brought to heel or defamed and potentially written out of the script.

6. Free Expression

Along with suppressing free thought, narcissists attempt to control what others express, particularly about them or things they believe relate back to them. Narcissists have trouble with the free expression of people around them for the same reason they are threatened by free thought. They feel compelled and entitled to exert their will over others to orchestrate a version of reality, no matter how distorted, that aligns with their needs.

COMING OUT OF DENIAL

As someone who has suffered violations at the hands of one or more narcissists, you have had your integrity and self-esteem targeted. The parts of you that come together to form and support you as an integrated, healthy person have been under attack. Particularly if the narcissist in your life has power over you in some way, you have been undermined, ambushed, and harmed emotionally and maybe physically. You may tell yourself it's not that bad and that real abuse and neglect are things that happen in other relationships or families, not yours. You may believe the narcissist is so important, special, or needy that s/he deserves a free pass. You probably blame yourself or feel responsible somehow for the narcissist's behavior, telling yourself what the narcissist always says or implies—that you are at fault and you need to change.

Denying reality can be a helpful short-term defense against overwhelming feelings.[3] Pushing away painful truths can give us a chance to process our fears and prepare us to face challenges. Denial is natural and even to some degree necessary in children growing up in narcissistic homes. It can shield us from realities we can't yet understand and help protect us from dangers we are not equipped to handle. But denial becomes a toxic form of lying when we allow it to paralyze us and use it to avoid taking appropriate action to protect ourselves and those we love. Long-term denial enables abusers and makes us and others vulnerable to further abuse. In time, denial becomes its own problem that keeps us stuck. Saying it isn't raining when it is does not keep us dry. It keeps us from taking shelter and staying warm. Others may look at us and wonder why we are ignoring that we are wet and cold. They may encourage us to come in with them to a place of safety and comfort. But until we end our denial and acknowledge the weather, we get wetter, colder, and more alone.

RECLAIMING YOUR RIGHTS

Even when we are actively confronting our denial, we may find it difficult to sort out what has happened and may still be happening to us. Narcissistically disordered people by definition project their own shame onto others; routinely blame others for their problems; and violate emotional, psychological, and physical boundaries. As someone who has been chronically shamed and blamed and had your boundaries crisscrossed, you are likely to be confused and plagued with self-doubt. You may feel, consciously or unconsciously, that you are somehow *less than*: less important, less deserving, less worthy, less good. You need some reminders about your intrinsic human rights, rights we *all* share.[4]

1. You have the right to your own thoughts and beliefs.
2. You have the right to disagree with others.

3. You have the right not to share your thoughts.
4. You have the right to express yourself freely.
5. You have the right to love and not love whom you wish.
6. You have the right to your own feelings.
7. You have the right not to feel what others feel or want you to feel.
8. You have the right to equal treatment.
9. You have the right to respectful treatment.
10. You have the right to advocate for your needs.
11. You have the right to advocate for your loved ones' needs.
12. You have the right to privacy and dignity.
13. You have the right to protect and defend yourself against attack.
14. You have the right to equal legal protection.
15. You have the right to personal safety and security.

If these rights sound like too much to expect, ask yourself why. Why don't you deserve these rights? Why does the narcissist in your life deserve them and not you? Why does the narcissist get to violate your rights?

RECOGNIZING THE NARCISSIST'S HYPOCRISY

Bottom line: Narcissists will always place their needs before yours. They have a *pathological disorder* that makes them different from neurotypical people. For the nondisordered, it is extremely difficult to comprehend narcissists' mind-set. They are riddled with hypocrisy and contradiction that make no intuitive sense to those who are emotionally stable.

The narcissist:

1. Is profoundly selfish but lacks a core self
2. Dismisses others' abilities and achievements and overestimates her/his own
3. Feels intense shame and readily shames and blames others
4. Is hypersensitive to slights and criticism while being hypercritical of others
5. Expects a free pass but is intolerant and unforgiving
6. Expects adoration but treats others with indifference or contempt
7. Demands loyalty and support but readily betrays and abandons

8. Demands control but accepts little to no responsibility
9. Is self-serving but expects generosity
10. Is disrespectful but demands special treatment

Narcissists' overcompensations for underlying emptiness and shame appear outrageous because they are outrageous. Their double standards are unjust and irrational, but make sense in their disordered mind. Narcissists' condition is pitiable but dangerous. Cognitively they are adults, but emotionally they are toddlers. Would you trust a toddler to understand your feelings, care about your needs, make decisions for you, or be a parent?

UNDERSTANDING YOUR ANGER

As someone who has been treated to narcissistic abuse, it is virtually inevitable that you feel anger. However, you may not realize you feel angry because the narcissist in your life has told you in countless ways that s/he is not accountable—that whatever you feel about her/his behavior is wrong, unfair, and your fault. You may feel confused and ashamed of your own anger because the narcissist has projected her/his anger onto you, saying that you are the one with an anger problem. Possibly you have sublimated your anger and turned it on yourself in the form of hypercritical self-talk and self-sabotage. You may have tried to drown it in alcohol, drugs, self-harm, gambling, shopping, and other compulsive behaviors. It is important to recognize that you feel anger and that your anger at the narcissist's abuse is appropriate and justified. Anger itself is not a bad thing. Anger is simply an emotion, and it has a rightful place in our lives. Anger can help us defend ourselves from attack and harm. It can embolden us to take needed action to protect ourselves and others and fight for justice.

But it is important to understand that the root of anger is a feeling of unfairness or harm. If you can sit with your anger and find the hurt and sense of violation driving it, you can begin to understand the full emotion and explore why you're feeling it. Although certainly anger in some cases can help us, it can also paralyze us or lead us on a destructive path that only creates more problems. Understanding the hurt—those feelings of unmet need—driving our anger helps us work with our emotions, not against them. Discovering what we really need is always the first step to finding a way to fulfill those needs.

UNDERSTANDING YOUR NEEDS

Food and water are needs. Love, belonging, safety, trust, and a sense of purpose are needs. Alcohol is not a need. Disordered eating is not a need. Compulsive sex is not a need. They are ways we try to soothe ourselves or control things that feel out of control. If we don't understand what we're feeling and what we need, often the ways we try to feel better or exert control are counterproductive and create additional problems in our lives. Often we do them to distract ourselves from the core issues we don't feel able to face. Like denial, seeking distraction is understandable as a way to alleviate pain. But escaping into distraction is a short-term fix that prolongs the unaddressed hurt and eventually adds to it. It prevents us from seeing ourselves and our situation clearly and blocks our ability to help ourselves get our needs met. Narcissists will always neglect our needs in favor of their own, and they may actively shame and punish us about our needs. But our needs do not go away, as much as we might wish and try to banish them. Needing means we are alive.

two

Identifying the Narcissist in Your Life

PERSONALITY DISORDERS CAN BE DIFFICULT TO DIAGNOSE FOR A PROFES-
sional; it can be pretty dicey to take it on yourself if you are not educated
in such matters. People's behavior and motives are complicated, and labels
are often simplistic and wrongheaded. Addictive behavior and depression,
for example, can resemble aspects of narcissism, and personality disorders
often coexist with those and other mental health problems. But realistically speaking, when it comes to pathological narcissism, an unprofessional
"diagnosis" may be all you are going to get.

WHY AN OFFICIAL DIAGNOSIS OF NPD IS UNLIKELY

Narcissism has the dubious distinction of more often being treated for
its traumatic impact on others than for the condition itself. As the saying goes, narcissism is a sickness for which everyone but the patient is
treated.

An official diagnosis of narcissistic personality disorder (NPD) frequently does not occur for the following reasons:

1. People with NPD are notoriously resistant to psychotherapy.
   The therapeutic process threatens their need to believe that they
   are infallible and above accountability. And it calls on them to do
   something they by and large hate: reflect on their own feelings and
   behavior. Thus, a great many narcissists never set foot in a therapist's
   office and as a result remain officially undiagnosed.

2. Narcissists who do pursue therapy often only do so to appease, at least temporarily, the demands of a spouse discussing divorce or a boss threatening the loss of a job. Sometimes narcissistically disordered people will seek therapy for help with depression or failed relationships. However, narcissists who experiment with therapy typically attempt to manipulate their therapist to support their delusions and/or quit to avoid the scary and painful work of self-reflection.[1]

3. Many therapists do not understand or recognize NPD (or the trauma that results from being around it).[2]

4. Clinicians who treat NPD oftentimes do not give an official diagnosis because of the stigma around it and the narcissist's intractability.[3]

It is important to note that some people struggling with NPD do stick with therapy.[4] Although there is disagreement about the efficacy of treatment, some therapists report degrees of success, and some narcissists themselves report becoming more self-aware and actively working on overcoming their distorted and reactive emotions and patterns of thinking and behaving. As with any serious mental health condition, pathological narcissism is something the person suffering with the problem must choose to work on. Loved ones can support the work, but the person with NPD must be motivated from within to change.

RECOGNIZING WHAT YOU'RE DEALING WITH

Having a narcissist in an important role in your life puts you at risk for significant if not devastating harm, and awareness is your best defense. People with NPD operate *unfairly* and *abusively*, with a toxic cocktail of infantile neediness and selfish disregard for the needs of others. You have likely been used, shamed, gaslighted, bullied, perhaps terrorized, and, adding to the craziness, told in endless ways that you are to blame for the abuse. The narcissist's abusive behavior is a cancer destroying your self-esteem, health, relationships, faith, and financial resources. However much you give the narcissist will never be enough, and what you hope to receive in return will not arrive.

Identifying who and what you are dealing with—the complexly insidious nature of NPD—is essential for disentangling yourself from the barbed wire that has been strung in and around your life. The diagnosis is for you, not them. You need it to

- validate your confusion and suffering;
- understand what you've been through and why;
- undo the narcissist's brainwashing influence;
- help others, such as children, in similar harm; and
- separate yourself from further abuse.

A WORD OF CAUTION

For those who have experienced narcissistic abuse, it may be tempting to confront the narcissist with your suspected diagnosis. But first consider your motives and the realities of the disorder. Has this person shown respect for your opinions, particularly if they are in any way critical of her/him? Is s/he open to self-reflection, personal accountability, or honest feedback? Has s/he demonstrated true concern for your feelings and needs? If the answers are genuinely yes, then you're probably not dealing with a narcissist. If the answers are no, telling the narcissist is likely only to elicit, at best, distorted pride or apathy, and at worst, vengeful rage. A common refrain from some narcissists is that other people are narcissists, and you may find your diagnosis projected right back onto you and broadcast to your family and social circle.

PART 2

NARCISSISTIC PERSONALITY DISORDER

three

Traits of Narcissistic Personality Disorder

NARCISSISM IS CONSIDERED A SPECTRUM DISORDER, MEANING IT EXISTS on a continuum, with some people exhibiting a few traits and others having full-blown narcissistic personality disorder (NPD). NPD is a Cluster B personality disorder, along with borderline personality disorder, antisocial personality disorder, and histrionic personality disorder. Cluster B personality disorders are characterized by dramatic, overreactive, and/or unpredictable patterns of thinking and behaving. NPD occurs in 6.2 percent of people, with greater numbers among men, 7.7 percent, than women, 4.8 percent. It has a high co-occurrence with other personality disorders, such as disorders relating to substance use, anxiety, and mood.[1]

NARCISSISM FICTIONS AND FACTS

Fictions

Here are some ideas about pathological narcissism that are false and potentially dangerous:

1. False: The roots of narcissism are vanity and self-love.
2. False: Being a narcissist means you're charming, smart, good-looking, and/or successful.
3. False: Only men are narcissists.
4. False: Narcissists are by nature great lovers.

5. False: Narcissists are masterminds with superior powers.
6. False: Narcissists can be cured by the right "empath" lover.
7. False: My narcissistic boyfriend/girlfriend will change for me.
8. False: If I make myself vulnerable, my narcissistic parent/partner/friend will trust me and open up.
9. False: Narcissists are evil geniuses who conceal themselves behind a charming exterior.
10. False: Narcissists really do care but just don't know how to show it.
11. False: Narcissists just need to learn humility.
12. False: Narcissists will respond to reason.
13. False: Narcissists make great leaders.
14. False: Narcissists are always scheming and looking for victims.
15. False: All therapists understand narcissism and how to treat narcissistic abuse trauma.
16. False: Narcissists cleverly hide their true identities.
17. False: Narcissists know they're narcissists.
18. False: Narcissists choose to be narcissistic.
19. False: Underneath it all, narcissists really do love their families and want the best for them.
20. False: Narcissists are obvious to spot.
21. False: If I leave my narcissistic spouse, the legal system will protect my kids and me.
22. False: Social media can make you a narcissist.
23. False: Narcissists don't have feelings.
24. False: Narcissism is untreatable.
25. False: We're all narcissists.

Facts

Here are some stark facts about narcissism that everyone should know:

1. Fact: Narcissistic personality disorder is a pathological and debilitating condition.
2. Fact: People with NPD lack a stable sense of identity and self-esteem.
3. Fact: Narcissists have an unrealistic view of people and relationships.
4. Fact: Narcissists have very limited or no emotional empathy for others, including their family members.
5. Fact: Narcissism is a coping mechanism based in shame.

6. Fact: Although some narcissists have the drive to become leaders, they do not operate for the greater good and tend not to support democracy.[2]
7. Fact: Narcissists habitually project their feelings onto others.
8. Fact: Narcissists are no smarter than anyone else.
9. Fact: People with NPD are ruled by self-doubt and shame but hide those feelings from themselves and others.
10. Fact: The narcissists' grandiosity and superiority are fragile defenses.
11. Fact: Narcissists typically lack self-awareness and avoid introspection.
12. Fact: NPD begins to form in early childhood.
13. Fact: Many of the world's most brutal dictators are malignant narcissists.[3]
14. Fact: Sadistic narcissists enjoy causing suffering and have no remorse.
15. Fact: Although narcissists can be quite calculating, they are primarily driven by unconscious emotions.
16. Fact: Narcissists may realize they are narcissistic, but they usually interpret that as a way of being special, not as a set of problems stemming from low self-esteem.
17. Fact: Some therapists do not understand narcissistic abuse and the complex trauma around it.
18. Fact: Narcissists often behave monstrously but are disturbed people, not monsters.
19. Fact: Narcissists view vulnerability as weakness.
20. Fact: If narcissists are not feeling threatened, they may be enjoyable to be around.
21. Fact: NPD occurs in both men and women, but is more common in men.
22. Fact: Narcissists do not treat others as they expect to be treated.
23. Fact: Narcissists lack moral integrity.
24. Fact: Narcissists feel justified when they hurt others.
25. Fact: Narcissists are incapable of unconditional love.

DEFINING TRAITS OF NARCISSISM

The American Psychiatric Association (APA) defines NPD as a condition characterized by pathological personality traits and impairments that show "a pervasive pattern of grandiosity (in fantasy or behavior), need for admiration, and lack of empathy, beginning by early adulthood and present in a variety of contexts."

According to the APA's criteria, published in the *Diagnostic and Statistical Manual of Mental Disorders*, 5th ed. (*DSM-5*),[4] a person qualifies for a diagnosis of NPD if s/he exhibits five or more of the traits in this list:

1. Is superior and grandiose
2. Has fantasies of unlimited success, power, brilliance, beauty, or ideal love
3. Believes s/he is special and should associate with high-status people or institutions
4. Expects excessive admiration
5. Has exaggerated entitlement
6. Is exploitative
7. Lacks emotional empathy
8. Is envious and believes others are envious of her/him
9. Is arrogant and haughty

Let's take a closer look at what the diagnostic criteria mean:

1. Superior and Grandiose

Narcissists adopt self-aggrandizement as a defense against underlying insecurity. They may be skilled at attracting, seducing, and influencing others to win praise and favor, but their grandiose superiority makes them abrasive and intolerant. They view others hierarchically as inferiors to be devalued, competitors to be beaten, or superiors to be won over.

2. Fantasies of Grandeur

Narcissists seek to inoculate themselves from fault by chasing an ideal of perfection. Needing to feel better than others to feel good enough, they have larger-than-life fantasies of invulnerability and omnipotence. Depending on their interests and strengths, they may dream of supreme achievement, intellectual prowess, unearthly beauty, and/or idealized romantic love.

3. Need to Feel Special

Narcissists derive their identity through the belief that they are special and should associate with other special, high-status people, causes, institutions, and the like, connections they lord over others in a campaign to further elevate themselves by devaluing those they view as competitors or underlings.

4. Admiration Seeking

Narcissists are well practiced at concealing their insecurity from others and themselves. But their profound underlying emptiness and shame are reflected in their correspondingly inordinate need for external validation. The term *narcissistic supply* refers to their compulsive use of others to feed their pretentious persona and placate their deep-seated feelings of inadequacy. Without admiration, narcissists experience destabilizing emotions, which can lead to deflation and depression. At home, they expect adoration without earning or returning it, often bullying family members into a habitual state of fear or guilt to get it and becoming enraged if the response appears tepid or feigned.

5. Exaggerated Entitlement

Because people with NPD must convince themselves that they are more deserving than others, to shore up their feelings of inferiority, they see themselves as entitled to special treatment and, without it, feel intolerably slighted. They expect more and better than what other people get and will not hesitate to make demands, lash out, cause a scene, play the victim, or sulk punishingly if "deprived." They insist on favored status and superior service, from the best table in restaurants to special deals at stores to the most attentive treatment at the doctor's office, salon, or gym. Being treated like a regular customer, whether in the world at large or at home, is impossibly demeaning and cause for resentment and retribution.

Narcissists' entitled belief system is further reflected in their tendency toward social intolerance and hierarchical political beliefs, including a disregard for democratic principles and a belief in authoritarian and/or military rule.[5]

 VIP TREATMENT

Travis and his family ate out and traveled a lot. His wife, Angie, said he always insisted on booking the best places, such as the Ritz Hotel when they went to Chicago. "He expected to be treated like an absolute king," she said. "Everybody had to bow to him or he would cause scenes and yell." Travis also was intolerant of noises and smells and would become enraged by electric fans, baby cries, or kitchen odors. "In restaurants he always expected the best table and would demand to be moved until he got it," Angie said. "It was the same thing in hotels. Wherever we stayed, he would insist on getting a different room at least once, and we'd all have to pack up and move our things." «

6. Exploitative

When it comes to relationships, narcissists operate without a moral compass, exploitatively with their interests foremost in mind. They use and manipulate others to manage their unstable self-esteem and rationalize their behavior, often abusive, to justify themselves. Individuals with NPD believe the rules do not apply to them and look to gain the upper hand in every situation.

7. Empathy Impaired

Perhaps the most outwardly harmful characteristic of NPD is a lack of emotional empathy. Although narcissists can usually cognitively recognize the perspectives of others,[6] they rarely connect emotionally with others' feelings and routinely hurt those around them to bolster themselves. As far as narcissists are concerned, other people, particularly family members, are extensions of themselves to be manipulated to meet their needs, which always take precedence.

Signs of empathy are
- good listening;
- reflecting back compassion and concern;
- validating other people's feelings;
- being willing to sincerely apologize and take responsibility;
- remembering and asking about others' lives; and
- acting on behalf of others' needs, even when it is inconvenient or difficult.

Consistent behavior to the contrary is a *narcissist alert*!

IT'S ALL ABOUT ME

Joanne had watched her mother die at the hospital the day before. She had been ill, but her death was sudden and surprised everyone. As Joanne was accompanying her father to his front door, her mother-in-law, who lived down the block and was walking by, launched into an angry diatribe about her car not starting. "She knew about my mother's death, but she went off about how infuriating it was to wait for a tow truck and what bad luck she was having, without saying a word to us about it," Joanne said. "We just stood there listening. Suddenly she interrupted herself and told my father, 'It's too bad about things.' She didn't say anything to me. Then she walked on, ranting about her car again. Dad and I just looked at each other in disbelief." ‹ ‹

8. Envious

Because they value appearances and superficial markers of worth and feel they deserve more than others do, people with NPD are prone to envy and the belief that others envy them. With an outsize sense of entitlement, they often actively covet what others have, whether material possessions, relationships, or achievements. When they see something as desirable, they are likely to go after it regardless of the consequences for others and, if thwarted, may try to sabotage or punish the person who has what they want. Because they view life competitively, they assume others are also trying to take what they have, which can lead to jealousy, paranoia, and false accusations.

9. Arrogant and Haughty

Narcissists continuously seek to elevate themselves, which drives them to rude, competitive, and explosive or punishing behavior, especially when feeling threatened or "crossed." They also are prone to ridiculing, bragging, gossiping, gloating, condescension, huffiness, "correcting," name-dropping, and/or making grand displays.

The Limitations of the APA's Criteria

Although the American Psychiatric Association's nine identified criteria for diagnosing NPD are a somewhat useful guide, it is important to understand the limitations of this list. Like any organization, the APA is a group of individuals with disagreements, biases, and political and financial agendas,[7] including pressures to comply with demands from the insurance industry. Many people in the field have decried the oversimplicity of the *DSM-5*[8] and pushed for a revision to the criteria for NPD and for personality disorders in general.[9]

A major criticism of the existing nine criteria for NPD is that they are too broad and open to interpretation.[10] Since a diagnosis can be made with five of the nine characteristics, two people labeled with NPD might only have one characteristic in common and therefore present with quite different personality profiles. Critics also fault the list for weighting all nine characteristics equally when in fact some are more salient than others. Many would argue, for example, that a lack of empathy is a more significant feature of NPD than being haughty or envious. Another problem cited is that the criteria for all four Cluster B personality disorders—narcissistic, histrionic, borderline, and antisocial—overlap in ways that often result in complicated and confusing "co-occurring diagnoses," such as NPD and BPD (borderline personality disorder), or NPD with APD (antisocial personality disorder) traits. Some psychologists find it more helpful to view the four disorders as different manifestations of the same underlying condition or as four dimensions on the same continuum.[11] An alternative dimensional model for diagnosing NPD, as opposed to the existing categorical one, was proposed in *DSM-5*.[12]

Perhaps the biggest criticism of the existing criteria, voiced by some leading psychotherapists who have direct clinical familiarity with narcissism, is that the criteria do not sufficiently address narcissists' internal state—the thoughts and emotions that drive their behavior.[13] The criteria also fail to fully acknowledge more closet (covert) expressions of NPD, which are just as debilitating as exhibitionist (overt) forms for people with the disorder, as well as for others treated to narcissistic abuses. Throughout this book, I explore these aspects of the disorder.

OTHER TRAITS OF NARCISSISM

In addition to the traits I've just described, there are other fundamental psychological aspects of pathological narcissism that are important to know to understand the condition.

Shame: The Narcissist's Underlying Emotion

Beneath narcissists' elaborate defense system is an emotionally unstable child driven by feelings of shame and unworthiness.[14] Missing the early developmental support to establish resilient internal love of self, the child fails to form mature capacities for self-reflection, emotional awareness, empathy, and love of others.[15] Instead, s/he overcompensates with claims of superiority and entitlement that s/he strains to assert through endless posturing. And s/he preemptively attempts to manipulate others to support her/his inflated self-beliefs and protect her-/himself from the shaming treatment s/he fears or may have come to expect.

As adults, narcissists walk a tightrope of self-deception, with their faulty emotional logic constantly tipping them off balance. Their defenses are artificial and unrealistic, but they must believe them to keep from psychological collapse and deflated depression. They need to feel superior to other people to feel good enough but are reliant on others for the validation they cannot give themselves. These tensions put them in constant conflict with their own impulses and with everyone around them, making for tumultuous relationships and love/hate attachments. In her insightful book *Stop Caretaking the Borderline or Narcissist*, Margalis Fjelstad describes the conflict:

> [Narcissists'] negative feelings are so intense that they try to push them away by projecting them onto someone else who is emotionally and intimately close, such as a child or a spouse. The [narcissist] has a desperate need to have someone else in his or her life to carry these overwhelming negative feelings, someone to accuse of causing the internal pain, someone to hate so as not to hate himself. This internal self-hatred is the real source of the [narcissist's] pain and anguish. [Narcissists] need someone to rescue them from these overwhelming feelings, to ease and soothe their fears. At the same time, they are afraid of being close to anyone . . . of being absorbed into someone else's personality and being annihilated, and they fear being used or humiliated by the person they depend on.[16]

Attention Seeking

Another common trait of NPD is an excessive need for attention, which narcissists depend on for psycho-emotional sustenance. Although we all have social needs, narcissists demand a level of attention beyond that of most neurotypical adults, often resorting to manipulation to get it. Narcissists figuratively suck all the oxygen out of the room. To gain attention, **exhibitionist narcissists** typically dominate socially, whereas **closet narcissists** use more passive-aggressive but equally insistent methods. Either way, they are vying for attention and a leg up. The narcissistic father, for example, may bitterly resent attention given to his own children and punish his spouse for it.

Emotionally Reactive

Because narcissists are overwhelmingly concerned with getting support for their grandiose self-beliefs to defend against interior vulnerability, they are hyperdefensive and emotionally reactive.[17] Their reactivity takes many forms, including haughtiness, huffiness, intolerance, blaming, and rage. The brittle and reactionary tendencies of people with NPD are exacerbated by their lack of emotional empathy, giving them license to routinely judge, hurt, and punish others.

Splitting and "Out of Sight, Out of Mind"

A defining feature of narcissistic personality disorder is a failure to internalize certain psychological milestones in childhood. People with NPD have two fundamental deficits that magnify their emotional reactivity and pathological treatment of others:

1. They experience mental splitting because they lack *whole object relations*.
2. They experience "out of sight, out of mind" because they lack *object constancy*.[18]

Whole object relations allows us to see ourselves and others in a fully integrated way as having both positive and negative qualities. Narcissists by definition lack whole object relations, which means they are unable to form a stable, realistic, and nuanced view of themselves and others. This psychological deficit means that they experience splitting, instead viewing people (or things) in opposite extremes as either perfect or worthless, all good or all bad, with little to no middle ground. Narcissists also lack **object constancy**, which is the ability to maintain an emotional connection with and positive feelings for people we care about in moments when we are physically apart from them or when they hurt or disappoint us. If a narcissist's child gets a bad grade, for example, the narcissist may react with anger, forgetting that the child is normally a strong and conscientious student. Both psychological deficits are believed to result from disrupted attachment to primary care-givers early in life.

Narcissists' lack of whole object relations and object constancy means that they constantly vacillate between idealizing and devaluing themselves and others and between emotional connection and disconnection. When narcissists are disappointed or angry with their partner, for example, their feelings about that person swing to contempt and rage. When they are physically apart from her/him, they experience "out of sight, out of mind" and struggle to maintain their emotional connectedness. This makes con-sistent, sustained trust and intimacy extremely difficult. Personality disorder expert Elinor Greenberg describes the problem this way:

> Most of the abuse of romantic partners occurs because the [narcissistic] abuser lacks Object Constancy and literally forgets that they care about their partner and all the positive history and good moments are now to-tally out of awareness. . . . When someone lacks this ability, it increases the likelihood that they will cheat on their partner.[19]

Vacillating Self-Concept

Looking at narcissists' internal experience, we find rigid and distorted self-beliefs that fluctuate between self-hatred and compensatory grandiose assertions of superiority and entitlement. Put another way, narcissists swing between deflated and inflated states of mind as they struggle to manage their self-esteem. They are highly dependent on others for the reassurance they can't give themselves, leading them to seek inordinate attention and admiration. Because their internal state is fragile and fluctuating and be-cause their defenses are built around the need to believe that they are special and privileged, they are haughty, arrogant, and oversensitive to criticism and slights. Their defensive coping mechanisms become abusive because of their poor self-awareness and lack of emotional empathy, which drive them to manipulate and punish others. For those treated to a narcissist's extreme neediness, demands for special treatment, and callous attitude, the experi-ence is draining and battering, like caring for an adult-size toddler armed with a nail gun.

Superficial Relationships

Given their myopic self-involvement, poor self-awareness, and fear of exposure, it is easy to understand why narcissists have superficial relationships. Their romantic partnerships tend to be short-lived exercises in giddy infatuation followed by harsh devaluation and possible discard. Narcissists, particularly men, often care more about the conquest than intimacy or lasting commitment.[20] Narcissists also have more tolerance for narcissism in others, with like attracting like.[21] Relationships or marriages that do last involve **codependent** and abusive dynamics. As friends, narcissists tend to be opportunistic and exploitative and have trouble sustaining connections over time. Both romantic partnerships and friendships are more likely to reflect expediency and mutual tolerance for dysfunction rather than shared concern and compassion. Psychotherapist and author of *The Narcissist You Know*, Joe Burgo described narcissistic friendship this way to HuffPost:

> In my experience, narcissists rarely have lasting friendships, but when they do, those friendships are best described as a mutual admiration society: 'I agree to support your inflated sense of self and you agree to support mine.' . . . These friendships can be quite stable and long-lasting provided that criticism is excluded and acceptance is unconditional. . . . True affection and real concern for one another are largely absent, and the attachment is fueled by mutual support for their narcissistic personalities.[22]

BAD BLOOD

Terry had long agonized over his father's harsh criticism of Terry's son David. David was a talented dancer who struggled with anxiety, and his grandfather regularly shamed him for not being "tough" and masculine enough. When David came out as gay, his grandfather wanted to send him to a conversion therapy school. "My father is off the wall, but this was too much. I told him no way," Terry said. At Thanksgiving, Terry and his family showed up at the country club where his parents and whole family had been eating Thanksgiving dinner together for years. "When we arrived, we were informed that we were no longer members of the club and were not permitted for dinner," Terry said. "My father had cut us out of the membership. I could see them sitting across the dining room. My brothers looked over but didn't get up. My parents ignored us. It was a shock, but I guess I should have expected it. We went home and made a huge taco dinner, which became a new tradition. My wife had been wanting to get out of the country club obligation for a long time. This was what finally pushed me to end contact with my father. I needed to stand up for my son." <<

 AND THE OSCAR GOES TO...

Isabel's mother, Stella, often went to outlandish lengths to get attention. At the dinner table one night when Isabel and her sisters and father were talking, Stella suddenly slipped from her chair and collapsed onto the floor, apparently unconscious. They rushed to her side and called 911, at which time she awoke. The same scenario played out a few more times. If the conversation shifted away from Stella, she would dramatically drop to the floor. Isabel said, "Pretty soon we knew that Mom's 'fainting spells' were more ploys for attention. After that, we ignored her and talked over it. She continued to fall sometimes. She'd lie there for a bit and then pretend to wake up in confusion." <<

THE NARCISSIST'S FEARS

Beneath the narcissist's larger-than-life persona are buried feelings of overwhelming fear. The narcissist has four primary fears that drive her/his defenses:

1. **Being Exposed** Whereas emotionally healthy people want to be "seen" by others and seek partners who are able to give them that recognition of self, narcissists attempt to conceal their faults and natural human weakness, both from others and from themselves. Ruled by insecurity and unable to recognize middle ground, narcissists are compelled to be "perfect" so as not to be exposed as hopelessly defective. Anything less than perfection, such as being ordinary or average, is the equivalent of worthlessness. Narcissists are threatened by anyone, typically a family member, who sees their flaws or fails to reflect back the version of themselves they need to believe in.

2. **Losing Control** Narcissists are truly the ultimate control freaks. Lacking a stable sense of identity and self-worth, they project an idealized image and work continuously to control that image and other people's perceptions of it. Their need for control is so intense that anyone in their sphere must also be controlled to sustain their self-beliefs.

3. **Being Humiliated** Narcissists experience any form of criticism, real or perceived, as a devastating loss of face. Being deprived of special status and treated like a "regular customer" represent an unbearable affront. Small meaningless slights, such as questioning something they've said or failing to give them acknowledgment, which others would easily brush off, can be cause for rage. Anything that stirs up feelings of vulnerability is tantamount to humiliation, which threatens their precious persona and triggers their **narcissistic injury**, or underlying shame. Narcissists are so afraid of humiliation that they may preemptively humiliate others to avoid appearing vulnerable themselves.

4. **Being Rejected** For people with NPD, any kind of rejection—personal, social, or professional—represents intensely invalidating evidence of their unlovability. Whereas healthy individuals will in time pick themselves up and try again after rejection, narcissists resort to all manner of twisted rationalizing, **hoovering** (drawing someone back in), and bitter reprisal to avoid intolerable feelings of not being good enough. Rejected narcissists may fight with their spouse for child custody not because they want their children but as a way to hurt their ex. They also may launch a calculated smear campaign to discredit that ex and thereby gain the upper hand in court, within their social circle, and with their kids.

Pity for the Narcissist?

Narcissists' fragility would arouse sympathy if not for their arrogant and often cruel lack of regard for other people's feelings, boundaries, and life struggles. For those of us with narcissistic family members or friends, feeling love and concern for them is normal. But it is vital to understand that narcissists do not care about their family's needs, most tragically those of their children and partner, unless those needs happen to align with their own.

THINGS NARCISSISTS DON'T DO

Narcissists play by different rules than the rest of us, with a double standard that means they expect special treatment in the form of benefits and exemptions. Just as they do things that are out of bounds for most of us, they also refuse to do things most of us do as a matter of course. Here are things emotionally grounded people do routinely, which narcissists rarely or never do.

1. Apologize

Admitting wrong is uncomfortable for most people, but the give-and-take in relationships at times calls for an acknowledgment of fault. Emotionally stable people usually know when they owe an apology and are willing to give it. Whether we interrupt, fail to deliver on a promise, say something hurtful, or lose our temper beyond reasonable bounds, we offer apology to show respect and caring.

Narcissists, on the other hand, never sincerely apologize. Seeing themselves as above reproach, they never feel they have done wrong. Their sense of superiority reinforces their belief that other inferior beings or unfair circumstances are always to blame for anything that goes awry, even (and especially) if the narcissists are actually responsible. When they express regret, it is for lost opportunities or misfortunes beyond their control, not their own choices.

Sometimes narcissists express a fake apology, or **fauxpology**, designed to pacify while deflecting responsibility back onto others. A fauxpology often begins with "I'm sorry you . . . ," as in, "I'm sorry you are so sensitive and thin-skinned" or "I'm sorry you can't let go of the past." They may also express regret, but not about something they have done.

2. Take Responsibility

Although narcissists are drawn to power, they repudiate responsibility. Because they have built their identity against fundamental feelings of worthlessness, they are intensely sensitive to shame and blame. Responsibility of any kind triggers narcissists' fear of exposure to criticism. They are so averse to responsibility that they systematically stage their life to avoid it and become highly adept at denying and projecting it onto others, particularly those closest within their sphere of power: their partner and children.

3. Self-Reflect

Narcissists are terrified of their own shadows—the long-hidden child within who was irreparably damaged and whose feelings of inferiority they constantly overcompensate for. For narcissists, self-reflection is dangerous territory to be avoided at all costs because it represents unbearable vulnerability and requires a level of emotional strength and awareness they never developed. This is why narcissists rarely seek therapy, and they avoid honest communication, refuse accountability, and readily resort to raging defensive outbursts and mind games to blunt the truth.

4. Forgive

For the same reason that narcissists do not apologize, they also never forgive. To them, everyone represents a potential threat to be defeated, and they are hypervigilant to perceived or (more rarely) real attack. Life is a battle zone, and narcissists are always fighting for their survival. They regard any kind of hurt as cause for retaliation and possible revenge. If someone apologizes to them (often in a misguided attempt to end conflict), they see it as proof of their righteous superiority and may take the opportunity to further punish that person for whatever s/he may or may not have done wrong. Genuine forgiveness is not part of narcissists' emotional lexicon, fundamentally because narcissists cannot forgive themselves.

5. Act Selflessly

Selflessness and altruism are the antithesis of narcissism. Because narcissists lack emotional empathy and have an inflated sense of entitlement, acting selflessly is beyond their comprehension. At their core, narcissists have little to give because they feel their survival is at stake and nothing else matters. Narcissists by definition are locked in an inward spiral of unmet early childhood needs and extravagant compensatory self-beliefs.

6. Express Real Feelings

When it comes to their feelings, narcissists hide, from others and from themselves. Narcissists lack the self-awareness to understand the underlying feelings that drive their behavior as well as the confidence to make themselves vulnerable enough to share those feelings. Narcissists operate competitively on raw survivalist instinct and are strangers to their innermost emotional realm.

7. See Emotional Nuance

Although they may be clever, particularly at manipulating people and spotting their vulnerabilities, narcissists lack an awareness of emotional nuance and are prone to simplistic black-and-white thinking. They tend to either idealize or devalue others, and project their own cynical emotional agenda, believing that others see life as they do—as a series of games or battles to be won. The wide continuum of emotion that healthy beings, especially the most empathetic, experience on a daily basis is lost on narcissists.

8. Show Gratitude

Gratitude is difficult for narcissists. They carry around feelings that life owes them things, they never have enough, and they always deserve more. They tend to look toward what they can get next and devalue what they have or, conversely, idealize what they have lost and dread what's next. It can make them hopelessly stuck, where they become frustrated and self-pitying victims in their own mind, fighting to defend their grandiose self-beliefs. When things go well, they attribute it to their own talent and superiority. When things go badly, they blame externalities.

9. Give Credit

As with showing gratitude, giving credit is very difficult for narcissists. Because of their extreme sense of entitlement and underlying feelings of deprivation, they feel fundamentally underappreciated and underacknowledged. Their craving for validation can make them ambitious, but it also makes giving proper credit to others next to impossible and taking unearned credit a constant compulsion. When other people, in particular family members, succeed, narcissists will typically ignore or undermine that success or attempt to take ownership of it somehow. If a narcissistic parent's child makes a varsity sport, for example, that parent is apt to brush it off or claim credit by saying something like "I taught her everything she knows" or "He got it from me."

10. Admit Vulnerability

Above all, narcissists avoid any display or suggestion of vulnerability. Intense insecurity drives their elaborate defensive posturing, and anything that triggers a feeling of vulnerability is overwhelmingly threatening and must be shut down. Although narcissists may feel self-pity and solicit sympathy, they do not reveal their deepest injuries and self-doubts, even and especially to themselves, if they can help it.

NARCISSISTIC "QUIRKS"

Looking beyond the narcissistic personality's classic traits, there are other things often mistaken for individual personality quirks that are actually fairly common and explainable aspects of pathological narcissism and NPD.

See whether you recognize these things in the narcissist(s) you know:

1. **They have food issues.** From having eating disorders, to overfeeding and fat-shaming their kids, to being stingy with food and stealing things off your plate, they have food issues relating to body image, shame, and control.
2. **They walk ahead of you.** They literally walk in front of you or way ahead because they're so impatient and/or need to show their kingly/queenly superiority.
3. **They have gift-giving issues.** Their self-centeredness leads them to
   - give or regift cheap or random things that show they have no idea or concern about what you like;
   - give you things they would want that you have no use for;
   - give excessively to show how thoughtful/generous/tasteful they are, particularly when trying to ingratiate themselves;
   - buy one for you and one for themselves; and/or
   - attach strings to your gift.
4. **They're conspiracy theorists.** Particularly closet narcissists view themselves as victims and project their envy, paranoia, and bankrupt motives onto others.
5. **They admire totalitarian leaders.** They respect dominance, view people hierarchically, and believe in an entitled class of superiors lording over the worthless masses.

6. **They don't answer questions directly.** This keeps you off guard while allowing them to avoid responsibility.

7. **They rewrite history.** They interpret events according to how they need to see things rather than as they are, and the past is open season for distortions, omissions, and outright lies.

8. **They speak in superlatives and hyperbole.** Having an all-or-nothing view of things, they tend to speak in exaggerated extremes, such as "best/worst," "terrific/terrible," and "perfect/worthless."

9. **They traumatize you before your important events.** Whether you're graduating, having an audition, celebrating a birthday, or getting married, they need to hijack your experience and sabotage you.

10. **They're name-droppers.** They name-drop to associate themselves with status, even if it's their second cousin once removed who met Madonna's ninth-grade teacher on a red-eye to Missoula.

11. **They sleep with and/or stay in touch with your ex.** Did your mother sleep with your boyfriend/girlfriend? Does your father have a "special" relationship with your ex-wife/husband? Did your ex sleep with your "best friend"? Lacking boundaries, this makes them feel superior and in control while humiliating you.

12. **They interrupt.** In particular, exhibitionist narcissists feel compelled to dominate the conversation; are easily bored because they miss nuance and lack empathy; have low impulse control; think they have more important things to say than you do; and believe they have greater entitlement to speak.

13. **They're poor sports.** When they win, they gloat because they feel superior. When they think they might lose, they cheat or may not play at all. And when they lose, they pitch a fit, pout, make excuses, or challenge the outcome because their self-worth is on the line.

14. **They manufacture drama.** Needing inordinate attention and lacking self-control and empathy for others, they overdramatize events, fuel conflict, and pry into other people's problems.

15. **They enjoy other people's suffering.** Their eager interest in and enjoyment of seeing others experience misfortune, known as *schadenfreude*, is linked to the envious and entitled belief that they deserve more and others deserve less.

16. **They're aggressive behind the wheel.** Their emotional reactivity and arrogance make them more likely to tailgate, speed, honk, drive on the shoulder, cross the center line into oncoming traffic, drive off-road, and experience road rage.[23]

OVERFEEDING AND FAT SHAMING

Liam was chubby growing up, and his mother frequently commented on his weight and discussed it with his father and friends. Liam had always blamed himself for overeating and felt ashamed of his body. But when his wife and son complained about his mother giving them huge portions at dinner and getting offended when they asked to serve themselves, Liam reexamined the past. "I realized that often as a kid I wasn't hungry when I ate. My mother had a terrible temper, and I was afraid she would get angry if I didn't eat," he said. "She always told me, 'Loving sons love their mother's cooking.'"

MAD AT THE WHEEL

Mike's parents often fought in the car, and his father would become enraged and scare the family by turning the radio up full volume and driving recklessly. "Once he slammed the brakes so hard, my face hit the seat and my nose broke," Mike recalled.

THE NARCISSIST ONLINE

Ah, the intersection of narcissism and social media. It's a match made in heaven, or hell, depending on how you look at it. Because narcissists survive and moreover thrive on attention, reaching innumerable people at the speed of light is irresistible. Social media make it easy for narcissists to present an idealized image of themselves and their life, as well as to play the lurking attack troll for sport.

Projecting Perfection

Users of social media by and large want to show a good face, but narcissists work overtime to garner attention and project enviable lives. Compared to others, they spend more time on social media, post more photos, especially selfies, and edit their photos more.[24] They may attempt to collect large numbers of "friends" and "followers" even if the vast majority are surface acquaintances or strangers. And they are likely to post images with signifiers of status to cultivate the perception that they are living the high life.

Using Others as Lifestyle Props

When narcissists post images of family members, those family members may appear more like lifestyle accessories or minor actors in a movie in which the image-poster is the lead. Narcissists' vanity often overrides other concerns, and as long as they look good, they may not care or may even enjoy posting images of their spouse, child, or friend that are awkward or unflattering. Conversely, narcissists may use social media to highlight their idealized partner, favored **golden child**, or high-profile friend. In that case, they may display their attractive mate or impressive friend, or may show off their golden child, emphasizing that child's activities, achievements, popularity, or cuteness/good looks. The **scapegoated child** may be shown in a less positive light or be conspicuously absent.

Too Much Information

Narcissists also are inclined to overshare or inappropriately bring their relationship, family, or friendship problems into social media public forums. Because they have little respect for boundaries, they are more likely than most to violate them online. Their emotional reactivity and competitive need to be right, to win, and to flaunt their superiority can lead them to act impulsively online, criticizing a spouse or ex or dragging their grievances about a community issue or local business into public view. Having an extreme need for attention and a distorted sense of entitlement, they are more likely to brag and otherwise display themselves ostentatiously. They are also more likely to use social media to embarrass, punish, and conduct smear campaigns about other people.

Online Trolling

Narcissists' rage and desire to dominate may also lead them to play the role of online troll, attacking community members or strangers with whom they happen to disagree or even just playing devil's advocate for the kick of it. Dominating and abusing others anonymously online can be addictive to narcissists, particularly closet narcissists, who prefer to keep their aggression and antagonism hidden.

ONLINE BULLY

Carol was a compulsive Facebook user who participated heavily in a local community forum. She had "enemies" and often got into disagreements with other forum members. When the forum administrators warned her about her combativeness, she began threatening legal action (she was a lawyer) against them. Eventually the administrators resigned, largely due to her ongoing antagonisms, and she leveraged an opportunity to take their place as an administrator. As a forum administrator, she immediately began dominating the conversation, stirring up controversy with innuendo and gossip, and attacking people who questioned her. When she began posting angry and self-pitying comments about her marriage, people began to quit the forum. Within three months, most of the members had moved to a new forum started by the previous administrators. Carol was allowed to join but was put on behavior probation, which she quickly violated, leading to her expulsion from the group. <<

NARCISSISTIC BOREDOM

We all feel bored from time to time, but narcissists often seem *inclined* to boredom and inattention, which quickly progresses into impatience and impulsivity. Narcissists tend to be easily bored, especially with other people, because they

- have a restricted inner life,
- have little genuine interest in others,
- need inordinate attention on themselves, and
- lack empathy for others' points of view or feelings.

Narcissists' continual vacillation between feelings of deficiency and overcompensating self-aggrandizement consumes their energy. Whether they are feeling worthless or on top of the world, they are obsessed with themselves. This constant self-focus, combined with their low to nil emotional empathy, disconnects them from and makes them indifferent to the feelings and perspectives of other people. Narcissists not only don't understand or much care about others, but regard others' needs as obstacles to getting the attention they feel they deserve. Other people bore and inconvenience them unless serving their need for validation.

Moreover, narcissists' primitive emotional intelligence and simplistic black-and-white thinking make them color blind to emotional complexity and nuance. Other people are more like silhouettes than detailed and dimensional beings. When others talk about themselves, narcissists find it tedious, if not infuriating. But when they are left alone, they face another kind of boredom: their own emptiness. What looks like fascination with self is myopic neediness. Their unmoored identity and lack of inner resiliency keep them dependent on others for the affirmation they cannot give themselves, or others. Ultimately this boredom with themselves and others makes *narcissists* boring—detached, rigid, predictable, single-minded.

Hand in hand with boredom is narcissists' preoccupation with the next new thing. Familiarity breeds contempt, and the grass is always greener somewhere else. Their own marriage, children, friendships, routines, and possessions rapidly lose their luster and fail to live up to narcissists' inflated expectations. Whatever club accepted them as a member is one they no longer want to be a member of. Reality disappoints, and the next great object of desire—a relationship, a job, a vacation, a car—is idealized. They believe that shiny object on the horizon will boost their self-esteem, reflect their true greatness, and fulfill their fantasy of perfection as all things before it have failed to do. This is why narcissists often place more value on the attentions and opinions of strangers or acquaintances than of their own family members.

Not all people with NPD walk away from commitment. Indeed, many stay in jobs and relationships. But intimacy and sustained attention on other people are all but impossible for them, and their long-term relationships are at best turbulent and alienated.

Causes of Narcissism and the Narcissist's Impaired Empathy

A S WITH OTHER PERSONALITY DISORDERS, THE ROOTS OF NPD ARE complex and most likely a mix of environment and biology.[1] No straightforward causal factor for NPD has been identified, at least in part because there are so many individual variables at work in child development. But consensus opinion points to insecure attachment with parents in infancy and childhood.

CAUSES AND DEVELOPMENT OF NARCISSISM

Children who develop NPD are believed to experience a fundamental disruption with primary caregivers that they attempt to adapt to by taking on narcissistic compensations. The disconnection may be the result of:

1. Inconsistent or negligent care
2. Emotional, psychological, physical, and/or sexual abuse
3. Persistent judgment or criticism
4. Fluctuations between idealizing and devaluing
5. Anxious smothering or overpraising
6. Rigid, superficial, or otherwise unrealistic expectations[2]

Such children receive the message that love and caretaking, which they need for survival, are conditional. Without adequately accepting, validating, and empathetic parenting, they experience disapproval for being themselves and/or approval for playing a role. They internalize a defining sense of shame while adopting a false self that may be rewarded by their parents. They fail to develop emotional empathy or a stable, realistic, and dimensional view of themselves and others and remain emotionally disconnected in their future relationships.[3]

Whether invalidated by a harshly devaluing narcissistic parent or indulged and overvalued for certain traits or abilities that differ from their true interests and personhood, people who develop NPD experience a fundamental division between their authentic self and their family culture. They work to hide their true nature, which causes them shame, and develop a substitute self to gain approval and/or avoid judgment.[4]

NPD occurs as a defensive adaptation in early childhood. If not properly addressed, it progresses in adolescence and becomes ingrained by early adulthood. Although it may become more pronounced and obvious in later adulthood, it does not arise then. Adults who seem to suddenly display narcissistic behaviors may be doing so because they have dropped their self-control with you, your view of things has shifted, or they are experiencing addiction or another form of mental illness that resembles aspects of narcissism. Similarly, normal developmental narcissistic behavior in childhood and the teenage years should not be mistaken for pathological narcissism and emerging NPD.

THE NARCISSIST'S IMPAIRED EMPATHY

It is often suggested that people with NPD have little or no empathy, but the reality is more complicated and calls for a closer look at how we understand and experience what we call empathy.

Three Types of Empathy

Contemporary psychology identifies three types of empathy: cognitive, emotional, and compassionate.[5] They might be best thought of together as dimensions of empathy because they are connected and build on one another.

Cognitive Empathy

Cognitive empathy involves identifying someone else's perspective and feelings. Drawing from our own experiences and observations and combining that understanding with what we know about someone else, we imagine their emotional state. We take their perspective without necessarily feeling their emotions or caring about them. Cognitive empathy can be abused when we use our understanding of someone's emotional state callously to manipulate or harm them.

Emotional Empathy

Emotional empathy involves feeling with someone else: the act of experiencing their emotions to a degree along with them. When we feel emotional, or affective, empathy for others, we imagine their perspective and allow ourselves to share in their emotion. It enables us to forge an emotional connection. Emotional empathy is derailed when we allow ourselves to get overwhelmed by it. When we are flooded emotionally by someone else's feelings or situation, we may react by shutting down or by becoming overwrought. Whether we are underreacting or overreacting, our own needs intrude and effectively block our ability to empathize emotionally. We fail to offer meaningful connection and potentially make things worse for the other person by shifting the attention away from them to ourselves.

Compassionate Empathy

Compassionate empathy combines cognitive and emotional empathy to take action to help if possible. We use our cognitive understanding and emotional connection to consider what might be helpful and attempt to provide that assistance where appropriate. Compassionate empathy can be very powerful in helping others, fighting for justice, and righting wrongs. It can go awry when we insert ourselves without being grounded in full understanding, genuine concern, or permission to help. If we overstep, we run the risk of alienating others, creating new problems for them, and/or potentially undermining their joy or adding to their pain.

Example of Healthy Empathetic Response

By way of example, we can imagine a father whose teenaged daughter has just failed an important test because she mistakenly misnumbered her answers. She knew the material but got a zero because her answers did not match correctly with the questions.

The father's first response is to offer *sympathy* to comfort his daughter's distress: "Sweetie, I'm so sorry. That's awful!"

Using *cognitive empathy*, he then thinks about how much she studied for the exam and what a conscientious student she is and adds, "You worked so hard to prepare. You always work hard, and you knew the answers."

As she begins to cry, he recalls a similar incident in his life. He shares *emotional empathy* as he tells her, "I had the same kind of thing happen to me on a math final. I wrote the wrong variable on each equation but did everything else correctly. It's so upsetting because you really do know the material, and the mistake seems insignificant next to how hard you've worked in the class." She asks him what he did about it, and he explains. "I asked my teacher to give me a chance to fix the error and show that I knew the material by doing extra credit. He allowed me to do an extra assignment and averaged the two grades together to bring my grade up to better reflect what I knew."

Finally, the father's empathy becomes *compassionate* as he explores how to help: "Your mistake was even smaller than mine. Maybe you should speak with your teacher. She's usually pretty understanding, right?" Calming down, his daughter says yes. He offers to talk with her teacher about it if she'd like him to. Cheered by his understanding and offer of help, his daughter tells him she'll talk to her teacher.

In this example, the father is able to connect with his daughter cognitively and emotionally and take appropriate compassionate steps to help. His initial sympathy quickly shifts to cognitive empathy and then emotional empathy, which builds into full compassionate action. He shows appropriate emotional attunement without becoming emotionally overwhelmed, which could have led him to underreact by shutting down or overreact by making it about himself. He offers constructive advice and assistance gently without overstepping, ultimately helping empower his daughter to handle the situation herself.

Example of Narcissistic Response

We can imagine the same scenario with a different father and teenaged daughter. When she tells him she failed an important test because she misnumbered her answers, he offers some sympathy and cognitive empathy: "Oh no! But you are such a great student. That's not fair!"

As she starts to cry, however, he suddenly feels uncomfortable with her emotion and unsure of what to say. He is tired from a hard day at work and resents having another problem to have to deal with. Annoyed, he says, "Okay, wait, calm down. Don't get hysterical."

She tries to explain how she's feeling: "Dad, I'm upset, not hysterical. I've worked hard in this class, and I knew the material."

A time when he failed a test flashes through his mind with searing embarrassment. He recalls his father berating him about it and feels angry that his daughter corrected him and doesn't recognize what an amazing dad he is. He makes a personal attack: "This is so typical, the pathetic crying like your mother! The two of you constantly burden me with your helpless routine!"

Hurt and overwhelmed, she yells back: "God, Dad, I'm not trying to burden you! I just feel upset!"

He continues, shaming her: "Let's just be honest here. You should have been more careful. You deserved to fail."

Enraged, he hurls his keys against the wall and storms out of the room.

Here the father responds initially with cognitive empathy, imagining his daughter's perspective after discovering she had failed an important exam she knew the answers to. But his consideration of her feelings quickly falters when he is faced with her tears. Instead of emotionally empathizing, he feels overloaded and becomes impatient and tries to shut down her feelings. When she tries to explain, he reacts with escalating anger. He projects his feelings of being burdened by her emotions when he says that she and her mother burden him and act helpless. Feeling ashamed about his own experience failing an exam and frustrated that he is unable to help his daughter, he projects again by blaming her for her problem. Finally, he lashes out with punishing violence and abrupt withdrawal.

EFFECTS OF THE NARCISSIST'S IMPAIRED EMPATHY

In this second example, the narcissistic father uses cognitive empathy to consider his daughter's experience of failing a test. But his empathy rapidly breaks down when his own feelings of fatigue, shame, and inadequacy intrude. His self-focus, unresolved feelings from the past, and lack of self-awareness override concern for his daughter and lead him to project and lash out at her. He fails to offer emotional or compassionate empathy, and he ends up using his cognitive empathy to hurt her.

It is often stated that narcissists simply lack empathy, but research and experience show us that they can display cognitive empathy, as well as emotional and compassionate empathy under certain circumstances, such as when they closely identify with someone and/or don't feel personally vulnerable or threatened. A 2014 article on empathy in NPD published by the American Psychological Association states that "there is growing evidence that individuals with pathological narcissism or NPD display significant impairments in emotional empathy, but display little to no impairment in cognitive empathy." The article further suggests that "individuals with pathological narcissism may be capable of processing affective [emotional] information, but don't *want* to engage in empathic processing so as not to lose control or appear vulnerable."[6]

For those treated to narcissists' irregular and dysfunctional empathy, what is most disorienting and disarming about them is their typical behavior pattern of seemingly turning their empathy on and off. Their ability to apply cognitive empathy to understand and predict the thoughts, feelings, and actions of others without consistently engaging in emotional or compassionate empathy is precisely why they can be so effective at manipulating, exploiting, and otherwise hurting those around them. If they did not recognize our feelings, likes and dislikes, strengths and vulnerabilities, they would have diminished power over us—little ability to influence our emotions either positively or negatively.

In relationship to the narcissists in our life, we proceed with the belief that because they appear to *see* us, they will also *feel* us, or care about our well-being. And as we empathize emotionally with their feelings, we naturally believe they will reciprocate and empathize emotionally with ours. Instead we meet the narcissists' limits like an invisible stone wall. Depending on our situation, we may spend years, even lifetimes striking that wall, blindsided and internalizing the narcissists' accusations that we are to blame again and again for the failed connection.

When we begin to consider that a narcissist is not operating with the same playbook as ours, we face an equally disturbing realization: The person we love does not love us back, at least not as we hope and need to be loved. It is horrible to keep trying and failing, but it is also horrible to confront the fact that no amount of trying will change the situation unless the narcissist we are close to takes the unusual step of seeking help to change and actively working on changing. When that person is our mother or father, confronting that parent's pathological selfishness is not only profoundly painful, it is also terrifying because it leaves us emotionally alone and un-parented in the world. For a child in particular, the existential threat of a parent not having the capacity to love us back is usually worse than accept-ing blame for that parent's neglect and abuse. If we are to blame, then we still have the possibility of doing something to fix the situation. If, on the other hand, our parent is intrinsically deficient as a caregiver, we have no agency to make things better, and our need to trust in a godlike figure who is protecting and guiding us is shattered. We face parentlessness, perhaps life's most difficult deprivation.

Although our dependence on parental caregiving diminishes in adult-hood, we continue to need parents, no matter how old we are. We may be mature and independent, we may have kids and grandkids, but we are always also children who look to our parents as guideposts throughout our lives, even after they have died. This is why it is so very difficult, even as we age and acknowledge our parents' sometimes epic flaws, to disengage from our need for glimpses of their decency and affection.

THE PERFECT EXTENSION OF ME

Rina was a talented singer and guitarist, musical ability she shared with her father. He subjected her to regular critiques, and before her auditions he would bring her to tears by pointing out flaws and insisting she be "perfect." To avoid his judgment, her mother took her to voice lessons secretly, and Rina began practicing her guitar privately with headphones. Feeling excluded, Rina's father became furious and complained that she was selfishly robbing him of his enjoyment of sharing their mutual love of music. Her mother said, "I tried to protect her and take most of his rage, but he would insult Rina, swear at her, and storm off. Usually the aftermath was that he would go into her room and have a two-hour 'discussion' about why she was wrong and he was right." <<

SPITEFUL BABY

Helena's troubles with her mother started long before she could talk. As an infant, she suffered an undetected neonatal stroke. Her mother, Maurine, said she was a colicky baby who was acting out to spite her. It wasn't until Helena lost her vision and partial facial muscle function at seven years old that an MRI identified her early stroke.

Following her loss of vision, Helena endured over two dozen surgeries and ultimately regained her sight. "My mother viewed my problems as competition, so she got sick a lot for attention," Helena said. "She never talked about my health or asked me how I was doing."

Helena said her mother abused her two younger sisters, but she was the primary target of Maurine's rage, both verbal and physical. Once when Helena brought home a report card of straight A's, her mother gave her a brutal beating, saying she should have gotten A+'s.

In their community Maurine couldn't do enough for other families. "Everyone loved her," Helena said. "She remembered everyone's birthday and baked them a cake. She was a Girl Scout leader. She'd take the girls on hikes and sew their uniforms. All of my friends loved her. No one noticed that my sisters and I weren't on the hikes. We never got birthday cakes."

Helena described her father as a narcissist, too, but she said he didn't target his kids as much as her mother did. "He was an alcoholic and a gambler, and he was gone a lot at work," Helena explained. "One of the most heartbreaking moments for me as a child was realizing Dad knew what was going on. After I got a bad beating from Mom, he brought me a candy bar."

Helena said one of the things that saved her while growing up was spending time with her grandparents. Her paternal grandfather would intervene on her behalf when her mother lost her temper. As a young adult, Helena interviewed members of her mother's family to try to figure her out. "It was immensely helpful to talk with them," she said. "I realized my mother's problems existed from a very young age, that it wasn't my fault."

These days, Helena has firm boundaries with her mother, including a 3,000-mile buffer between them. She says her mother hasn't changed much, describing her most recent visit with Maurine: "My 22-year-old daughter is very pretty and often gets looks. We took my mother out for dinner one night, and some young men at a nearby table noticed my daughter. They were smiling and trying to catch her eye, something my daughter dislikes and tried to ignore." On the car ride after dinner, Maurine would not stop chuckling. Helena said, "Mom had a familiar smug look on her face. When I finally asked her why she was laughing, she said, 'I've still got it, the sex appeal. Did you see those good-looking men staring at me?'" Helena continued, "My mother is almost 80 and has facial paralysis and one eye sewn shut."

Helena said, "I've tried hard to have a workable relationship with my mother, not a loving one. She doesn't have a clue what that is. I've never had a single moment of maternal affection from her." <<

five

Closet, Exhibitionist, and Malignant Narcissism

A S A SPECTRUM DISORDER, NARCISSISM OCCURS TO DIFFERENT DEGREES, from a few narcissistic traits to extreme NPD. It also occurs in somewhat different forms, including closet, exhibitionist, and malignant.

CLOSET NARCISSISM VERSUS EXHIBITIONIST NARCISSISM

Often people talk about overt and covert narcissism, with overt referring to openly grandiose and domineering behavior and covert referring to less obvious self-importance and manipulation. But there are additional distinctions between these two expressions of pathological narcissism and NPD that are important for identifying their typical behaviors and the underlying emotions that give rise to them. To be more precisely descriptive, I use the terms *exhibitionist narcissist* and *closet narcissist*, which were originally coined by psychiatrist and personality disorder pioneer James L. Masterson.

Both exhibitionist and closet narcissists have the same fundamental problem with unstable self-esteem and an unmoored sense of identity, and both have grandiose compensations for their shame and insecurity. Both also have rigid and distorted thinking patterns, lack self-awareness and emotional empathy, and fail to see themselves and others in a whole, nuanced, and realistic way. But while the exhibitionist narcissist dominates conversations and basks in the limelight, the closet narcissist finds that level of attention uncomfortable and potentially threatening. According to Dr. Elinor Greenberg, "usually [closet narcissists] have experienced early and persistent humiliations, which have made them feel extremely conflicted about being in the spotlight."[1] Although some characterize closet narcissists as simply introverted, their reticence is not necessarily due to natural introversion; rather, it is because in the culture of their family it was dangerous to openly seek attention. This also left them unable to "mobilize a defensive grandiose facade" as the exhibitionist does.[2] This is why they are sometimes referred to as *vulnerable narcissists*. They still have the "I am special" defense but look to an idealized other, perhaps a kind of stand-in for their overbearing exhibitionist narcissistic parent, to demonstrate their specialness through association. Closet narcissists see themselves as exceptional, then, through their connection to people, institutions, systems, causes, and the like that they idealize and derive a feeling of status from. They may seek out mentors or forms of authority and serve diligently and efface themselves with those they admire.

Because they fear failure and exposure, closet narcissists are also apt to defer decisions to others, avoid direct confrontation, and use indirect means to get what they want. They are afraid to own their opinions and feelings, while also being prone to disappointment and rage when their needs are not divined by those close to them. They can be just as haughty, unforgiving, and demanding as exhibitionist narcissists but tend to express their sense of entitlement in quieter, less direct ways. They prefer to draw attention and exert control by playing on sympathies, using guilt, and making passive-aggressive maneuvers. Craving power but too fearful to take it, they embrace the role of victim and use that to justify their mistreatment of others. As victims in their own mind, they are prone to harbor resentment and envy, play the martyr, experience paranoia, and use underhanded means to manipulate and punish. Because of their more hidden nature, closet narcissists are often harder to identify as narcissists, and their grandiosity, anger, and callousness may more easily go under the radar with others. They frequently cultivate a self-sacrificing do-gooder persona in their social and/or professional circles that belies their ruthless self-interest and abuse of family members.

By contrast, exhibitionist narcissists typically rely on extravagant displays to scaffold their shaky ego. They seek to elevate themselves by drawing admiring attention and dominating through whatever power is at their disposal—charisma, intelligence, connections, wealth, physical strength, good looks, and so on. They make no secret of their competitive drive to outshine and outdo others, and they will humiliate and otherwise punish those who question or threaten their superiority and entitlement. They, too, seek out status by association, but they do not place themselves in subservient or adoring roles because they believe that they are already perfect and there is nothing anyone can teach them. For the same reason, they tend to refuse help and may eschew victimhood, viewing that as weakness and a loss of face.

Exhibitionist narcissists' (false) bravado and larger-than-life personalities can be impressive at first, especially to closet narcissists who long for the brash confidence exhibitionists appear to have. They may seem powerful, self-possessed, even invulnerable, qualities that can land them in positions of authority and institutionalized power and in extreme cases lead to large-scale, catastrophic abuses, such as genocide, religious persecution, and environmental holocaust.

But whether they are bold bullies or shrinking violets, aggressive or passive-aggressive, both exhibitionist and closet narcissists have fragile defenses that are dependent on external validation. Both are prone to idealize and devalue, seeing others as either perfect or worthless and punishing and/or rejecting those who inevitably disappoint.

General Narcissistic Traits

Both exhibitionist and closet narcissists:
1. Are hypersensitive to perceived and real slights
2. Are indifferent or callous to the feelings and needs of others
3. Have delusions of grandeur
4. Expect special treatment
5. Are intolerant of criticism
6. Rarely or never genuinely apologize or take responsibility for their actions
7. Derive self-esteem from associating themselves with high-status things, people, institutions, systems, or causes/beliefs
8. Target others who deprive them of what they believe they deserve
9. Distort reality through gaslighting

10. Triangulate to control and undermine communication
11. Divide and conquer others for leverage
12. Compulsively scapegoat and idealize others
13. View life in simplistic binary terms—good/bad, perfect/worthless
14. Are preoccupied with appearances
15. Overestimate (and underestimate) their importance and abilities
16. Categorize others hierarchically as inferiors, superiors, or competitors
17. Fluctuate between inflated self-aggrandizement and deflated depression
18. Project their own feelings and behavior onto others
19. Lack self-awareness and avoid introspection
20. Have superficial and exploitative relationships
21. View vulnerability as weakness
22. Routinely violate boundaries
23. Overreact to disappointments
24. Demand perfection
25. Lack interest in things regarded as irrelevant to self
26. Objectify others
27. Become easily bored and annoyed when attention is directed away from them
28. Are prone to defensive rage
29. Believe their opinion is the only legitimate one
30. Expect others to know what they want/need

Exhibitionist narcissists are also prone to:
1. Compulsively attract attention to themselves
2. Make dramatic, loud, or otherwise ostentatious displays
3. Act outwardly arrogant and haughty, especially with those they view as underlings
4. Demand admiration and agreement and without it react with impatience or rage
5. Become confrontational and combative when angered
6. Engage in rages far beyond normal anger
7. Make scenes and throw public tantrums
8. Appear charismatic in public settings while being negligent/abusive at home
9. Avoid appearances of vulnerability and refuse help

10. Preen and brag
11. Listen poorly and interrupt often
12. Lecture and interrogate
13. Need to feel expert at everything and like to give advice
14. Rarely acknowledge or credit others, and try to "own" others' talent and success
15. Bolster themselves by besting and devaluing others
16. Need to feel perfect and view anything less as failure

Closet narcissists are also prone:
1. Control with silent treatment, stonewalling, and other forms of withholding
2. Manipulate through guilt and self-pitying performances
3. Flatter and fawn over others to win favor
4. Feign innocence
5. Humblebrag
6. Behave worshipfully and go beyond the call of duty with people they idealize
7. Have delusions of victimization and persecution
8. Appear insecure or anxious and ask for help or advice
9. Stage a crisis to gain attention
10. Take pleasure in others people's problems and tragedies
11. Harbor long-term grudges
12. Resist answering questions directly
13. Exaggerate suffering and sickness to garner sympathy
14. Blame problems and failures on "unfair" people, institutions, and circumstances
15. Use backhanded tactics, such as gossip and smear campaigns, against people they envy
16. Criticize indirectly through implied blame, lack of acknowledgment, and unfavorable comparison

It can be very helpful to identify these two different manifestations of NPD, but it is important to keep in mind, when you're trying to make sense of the madness, that across these categories there can be gray areas and overlap. Very little in human nature, or nature at all, is clear-cut. In my experience, people with pathological narcissism and NPD tend to be primarily exhibitionist or closet, but they may have some traits from both types. Similarly, when we look at personality disorders more generally, we typically see overlap among types rather than absolute expressions of each type.

MALIGNANT NARCISSISM

Virulent and dangerous, malignant narcissism is an extreme expression of NPD. Although it is not an official diagnostic category, many psychologists view malignant narcissism as a hybrid disorder of narcissistic and antisocial traits, including aggression, paranoia, and sadism.[3] However malignantly they behave, all people with NPD struggle with underlying shame and feed their insufficient self-esteem with self-aggrandizing compensations. Nonmalignant narcissists *prefer* to moderate their self-esteem without being openly combative, and resort to attack as a secondary strategy when they feel threatened, diminished, or disillusioned. Malignant narcissists, on the other hand, meet their needs *primarily* through exploitation and dominance, which may include emotional, psychological, physical, and/or sexual violation.[4]

Malignant narcissists are most commonly exhibitionist but are sometimes closet.[5] Exhibitionist malignant narcissists constantly assess social hierarchies and demand absolute control. Prone to paranoia and envy, they savagely devalue others to feel superior and take down anyone or anything they view as an impediment or threat. In the case of closet malignant narcissists, they are more likely to keep their venomous impulses and savage behavior on the down low, using less conspicuous strategies to dominate and defeat anyone they regard as an enemy or even a mere obstacle. Their preference for keeping a low profile can lead them to be Machiavellian in their pursuit of social dominance.

Malignant narcissists often have sadistic inclinations but are not necessarily full-blown sadists. Although malignant narcissists may enjoy willfully inflicting suffering or humiliation on others, their primary motivation, as is the case with all people who suffer from NPD, is to drive away deep-seated feelings of defectiveness.[6]

Malignant Narcissistic Traits

Here are additional characteristics often seen in the malignant narcissist:

1. Routinely ridicules and humiliates others in games of one-upmanship
2. Studies a group for the most vulnerable and attacks to display dominance
3. Flouts rules and codes of conduct
4. Views weakness with ruthless contempt
5. Isolates others from social support
6. Engages in impulsive and calculated destruction
7. Violates personal boundaries, social norms, and taboos
8. Uses coercion and punishment to overpower others
9. Intimidates with threats, interrogation, and terror
10. Enjoys making others suffer
11. Exploits positions of authority to suppress discord or dissent
12. Justifies violent behavior for personal ends

six

Narcissistic Abuse

A S A SPECIES, HUMANS HAVE A REMARKABLY CONSISTENT AND SHARED sense of fairness. We recognize it when we see it, and when we don't, we may feel frustrated, disgusted, even outraged and driven to action. Similarly, most of us try to abide by a moral code in our dealings with others. We may fail along the way, but more often than not we try to follow the Golden Rule: *Do unto others as you would have them do unto you.*

Although we begin to try to teach our two- or three-year-olds the concept of the Golden Rule, we do not expect children of that age to be able to act on it consistently, if at all. That is because they are not emotionally and psychologically developed enough to see much beyond their own immediate needs. But over time, emotionally healthy parents come to expect their children to learn and demonstrate fair play and compassion for others. Controlling our impulses, recognizing other points of view, and respecting other people's feelings are hallmarks of maturity and emotional intelligence. Without those skills, we lack empathy, and when we lack empathy, we lack the capacity for acceptance and love—love of self and love of others.

As we have learned, individuals with NPD are emotionally stuck at a young child's developmental level. Deprived of adequate nurturing, children who form narcissistic adaptations are unable to develop a stable sense of self-definition and self-worth, a profound lifelong impairment. While they continue to develop in other areas, they remain emotionally stunted and unsure of their place in the scheme of things. Lacking a secure identity, they look to others to define themselves and stabilize their dysregulated self-esteem, using people around them without regard for those individuals' needs or the harm they inflict in attempting to get their own needs met.

Having gotten this far as a reader, you know just how absurd the Golden Rule sounds in the context of narcissism. For the person with NPD, the Golden Rule is turned on its head into something like this:

> *Do unto others as I would never allow them to do unto me because I am better and more deserving, and by the way I need you to tell me and show me that I am superior and entitled 24/7 because I am deeply afraid I'm really not, and if you don't give me what I demand right now, I'll punish the hell out of you into perpetuity.*

Unless they are malignant types, those with NPD do not necessarily set out to hurt other people. Usually they are caught up in their own distorted thinking patterns and trying to manage their shaky self-esteem. But their combination of traits inevitably leads to abusive behavior that is doled out habitually to the people around them. In this very real sense, narcissists are by definition abusers who do harm to others as a matter of course.

NARCISSISM IS AN ABUSIVE DISORDER

Narcissists certainly aren't the only type of people who lack empathy. But it is their lack of empathy coinciding with a competitive sense of superiority, inflated entitlement, low self-awareness, and constant need for admiring attention that makes them so very toxic. They aren't just insensitive and selfish, arrogant and devaluing, manipulative and exploitative. They are also *endlessly demanding.* They want attention. They want approval. They want admiration. They want agreement. They want everyone around them to validate their distorted self-serving reality and continuously hold up a mirror reflecting that false reality back to them as if it were irrefutable fact. They want to mistreat others with impunity and be told they are wonderful while doing it.[1] For those on the receiving end of such expectations, it is nothing short of crazy-making torment. Narcissists expect you to:

1. Give without expectations of receiving in return
2. Listen without being heard

3. Respect their boundaries while ignoring your own
4. Agree and acquiesce without question
5. Accept their distortions as facts
6. Support their belief that they are superior to you
7. Endure condescension, belittlement, and rage without complaint
8. Cater to their needs while sacrificing your own
9. Serve their privilege over yours
10. Take responsibility for how they are hurting you

Dr. Elinor Greenberg explains, "It is literally impossible for people with narcissistic personality disorder to not eventually emotionally abuse whomever they are with. They simply lack the basic capacities that would prevent that—whole object relations, object constancy, and emotional empathy. And no matter what they promise their new romantic partner, they cannot simply change without years of appropriate psychotherapy and a lot of hard work."[2]

BEHIND THE MASK: THE BULLY, COWARD, LIAR, AND FRAUD

It's not nice to call names. But when it comes to people with NPD, calling them out is a matter of survival for those dealing with their abuse, as well as for those who don't understand the extreme harm they do. All narcissists wear a mask, or false persona. And if you stripped away the mask, you'd find vulnerability that would be pitiable if it weren't so petty and vicious.

But chances are, you won't ever remove a narcissist's mask, because s/he defends it at all costs with a full arsenal of preemptive, controlling, and combative tactics. The narcissist is in essence an emotionally primitive child with an adult savvy for manipulating and exploiting.

The Bully

Narcissists are classic bullies. They bluster, ambush, attack without cause, and prey on the most vulnerable, usually those who love and depend on them, namely their partner and children, who as a result carry lasting trauma. Narcissists often also bully susceptible friends, neighbors, employees, and "underlings" in their path, such as waiters and clerks. Exploiting their power over others feeds their need to feel superior, and their lack of emotional empathy and sense of entitlement give them free range to abuse without the troubling hindrance of a conscience.

The Coward

Narcissists are fundamentally terrified of themselves and anyone who might see through their mask. Their driving motivation is to shield themselves from threatening emotions that trigger their buried sense of worthlessness, or narcissistic injury. They avoid self-reflection, refuse accountability, and rationalize their own abusive treatment of others. Often they strike and run, initiating surprise attacks and retreating before being confronted with the consequences of their rage. Narcissists also may behave passive-aggressively, cloaking their rage in self-pitying performances meant to induce guilt and blame. Whatever hurtful tactics they use, narcissists rarely if ever take responsibility for what they say and do. Instead they deny their abuse and project it onto others, most often those they have abused, further exacerbating the harm they do.

The Liar

Narcissists are the worst kind of liars—those who lie to themselves and demand that others support their self-deceptions. They continuously attempt to control others' perceptions of them, and when they can't, they resort to nasty and often violent reprisal. The narcissist may cast herself as a highly principled person, but in reality she is only concerned with her own needs and is too vulnerable and rigid-minded to face life's complex realities, especially those that threaten her elaborate defenses. She may talk a good game, but when it comes to facts and truth, she deflects, dismisses, stonewalls, and blames others. The narcissist may, for example, rage at her son for getting an A- grade instead of an A, because she feels threatened by her son's academic success, she is angry about a fight she had with her spouse, or she is projecting a self-centered expectation of perfection.

The Fraud

People with NPD struggle with a fundamental impostor syndrome, hiding their underlying insecurity behind arrogant privilege. They exaggerate, brag, and take unearned credit to bolster their self-esteem and may go to great lengths to create appearances of being caring and noble while mistreating those closest to them. They have superficial relationships and are incapable of authentic intimacy or selfless giving. They pretend at love, parenting, friend-ship, and any other important relationships in life. If they are idealizing you or attempting to win your admiration, they may mimic exemplary behavior, but their motives are self-centered, and their idealization is a projection that will be followed by devaluation when they become bored and disappointed.

PATTERNS OF NARCISSISTIC ABUSE

Those intimately familiar with narcissists know too well their emotionally, psychologically, and in some cases physically and sexually abusive actions, which may surface day to day, hour to hour. To anyone experiencing such treatment, people with NPD, especially those on the malignant end of the spectrum, often seem monstrous. They cause extraordinary trauma, partic-ularly in the lives of those closest to them, with little to no remorse but instead the belief that their behavior is reasonable and justified. Targeted family members may experience extreme forms of assault to their mind and body. Codependent partners and children in such circumstances may be preyed upon with systematic violations for years, while being told in count-less ways that they invite the abuse and deserve what they get.

Although like anyone narcissists have different histories and personali-ties, their abusive behavior manifests in remarkably consistent ways, includ-ing the following patterns:

1. Refusal to take responsibility
2. Projection of abusive behavior and selfish motives onto others
3. Baiting, ridiculing, and humiliating (often presented as "teasing") to gain an advantage and feel superior
4. Hypersensitivity to slights and criticism
5. Pitting people against one another (a.k.a. divide and conquer)
6. Endlessly demanding of agreement and admiration
7. Inability to share attention with others, even their children
8. Sudden, often violent rage with a hurricane's ferocity
9. Scapegoating "loved" ones
10. Berating and bullying
11. Gaslighting (making you think you're crazy)
12. Entitled, arrogant abuse of "underlings," such as employees, wait staff, clerks, and secretaries

13. Grandiose assertions of superiority and omnipotence
14. Indifference, impatience, and/or anger with others' illness, loss, and misfortune
15. Dismissal and denial, often outrageous in the face of blatant truth
16. Calculated charm on the surface and appalling treatment of family members behind the curtain

Hidden Trauma

Those unfamiliar with NPD and narcissistic abuse typically find it incomprehensible. This is because the narcissist's lack of a moral compass is difficult to imagine without direct experience with it and because people with NPD generally work to present a picture of normalcy or even an ideal "perfect" life to outsiders. Even many therapists are unschooled in NPD and its damage to those who live with narcissists, which frequently leads to post-traumatic stress disorder and a host of other lasting emotional and health effects.

Exhibitionist narcissists are often publicly charismatic, perhaps even heroic, making their family's experience of neglect and abuse invisible to others. Closet narcissists are expert at keeping their pathology hidden in the shadows, often presenting themselves as great humanitarians, devoted family members, or wronged victims, with outsiders unaware of their morally bankrupt behavior behind the scenes.

Thus, those harmed by narcissistic abuse are further traumatized by the isolation and self-doubt that come with it. And they are vulnerable to judgment and ill-conceived advice from outsiders who don't understand and may encourage them to forgive, confront, or reconcile with the narcissist and in doing so open themselves to further abuse.

Torture: Coercion, Punishment, and Sadism

As the saying goes, we often hurt the ones we love. But narcissists, particularly more malignant ones, torture others, often deliberately and with little to no restraint or remorse. If that sounds like hyperbole, let's look at Merriam-Webster's definition of *torture*: "the infliction of intense pain to coerce, punish, or afford sadistic pleasure" and "anguish of body or mind." Anyone who has had the misfortune of being targeted by a narcissist knows very well that *torture* is in fact precisely the word for the experience. The abuse can range from psycho-emotional to physical and sexual, but it is *inevitable* because narcissists feel justified when they hurt others, while at the same time they are always attempting to exert control.

Coercion

"Coercion" is the first part of the dictionary definition of *torture*. Narcissists coerce others, especially their family members, to uphold the manufactured identity they create for themselves in place of the insecurity they actually feel beneath their assertions of superiority. They constantly work to convince themselves that they are perfect (i.e., not flawed), and they resort to all means of coercion to exact cooperation from those around them to support their need to feel exceptional, extraordinary, and invincible.

Here are common coercive tactics narcissistically disordered people use, unconsciously and consciously, to gain compliance from others.

1. **Isolation:** removing the target's independence, such as by restricting contact with friends, outside family, and social connections; constraining physical freedom; and limiting financial resources

2. **Removal of Free Will:** destabilizing the target's fundamental sense of self, reality, and worldview through persistent questioning and negative judgment

3. **Instilled Powerlessness:** undermining the target's confidence in her/his thoughts, feelings, and perceptions through distortions of reality, gaslighting, and dismissing and denying truths and facts to cause self-doubt and **cognitive dissonance**

4. **Thought Control:** controlling acceptable opinion and expression in the target through interrogation, judgment, intimidation, rejection, and unspoken rules of engagement

5. **Terror:** controlling the target's words, actions, and thoughts through implied, threatened, or real verbal, physical, and/or sexual violence, often combined with intermittent repentance, promises of change, and/or rewards to keep the target "in the game" and holding out hope for change

Punishment

"Punishment" is the second part of our dictionary definition of *torture*. Narcissists are not capable of sustained love, loyalty, or respect for others, even and often especially those who in fact love and are loyal to and respectful of them. Anyone who triggers, usually inadvertently, their profound insecurity, or narcissistic injury (that early childhood psycho-emotional wound), is fair game for a host of punishments. Narcissists punish for numerous reasons, and they do it without remorse, believing others deserve it and would do the same to them if they were clever enough and given the chance.

Narcissists punish to:

1. Obtain/regain compliance
2. Demonstrate their powers of influence
3. Get revenge
4. Vent their rage
5. Assert their entitlement
6. Shut down potential or actual threats
7. Defeat "competition"
8. Display their dominance
9. Get "respect"
10. Create fear
11. Derive sadistic pleasure

Sadism

Here we come to the third part of our dictionary definition of *torture*: "sadistic pleasure" in pursuit of causing "anguish of body or mind." Malignant narcissists are often sadistic, experiencing pleasure, frequently sexual, through torturing others. They aren't hurting others just because they lack a conscience and are trying to moderate their self-esteem. They are doing it also because they enjoy and even delight in humiliating and dehumanizing others. People with NPD are not necessarily sadistic, but the ones who are make criminally monstrous abusers who will torment those they are meant to love.[3]

 FAMILY TRADITION

Melody's first memory, at three years old, was of her father beating her across the face with a belt. On that day, Sean, five, was trying to protect his younger siblings from the beating by hiding them in a closet. But, in time, Sean's protectiveness gave way to abusive behavior of his own. "The good was beaten out of my brother. He was like monkey-see, monkey-do with our father," Melody said. Soon, Sean began raping and beating Melody.

In addition to her father's physical abuse of the kids and his wife, there were his continuous psychological assaults, except on Brian, who was the family golden child. Melody recalls her father constantly saying her only worth in life was as a "whore." He groped her and removed the door to her bedroom so he could watch her undress. Then, he would put the door back on and remove the knob to trap her inside. Melody said, "I would pound the door and cuss to be let out. Mother knew all this was going on. She would say, 'Would you rather be in a foster home?' She called Sean's physical and sexual abuse of me 'a normal outlet for him.' I tended to think of Mother as more benign, but after Father died, I realized she used him to be an abuser by proxy. She was just as sadistic. She thrived on it like oxygen."

Looking back, Melody realizes she is the only one in her family who got out without having her spirit crushed and becoming an abuser herself. "I fought like hell. I never gave up my core values. My mother could manipulate my brothers, but she didn't know what to do with me. I refused to accept when my parents told me no one would love me. When my father told me I was ugly, I thought, 'I came from you so *you* must feel ugly.' I didn't have a name for it then, but I figured out it was projection."

Melody said her brothers haven't fared as well. In their 40s, both still live at home with their mother and continue the violent family tradition by abusing their girlfriends. Sean hasn't had a job in years, and Brian "lives like an entitled king," with an expensive car collection. "Brian kicked Mother out of the master bedroom and took over half of the house. It's like sadomasochism with them. Both my brothers think they'll get the house when she dies," Melody said, and then added, "Mother hollowed them out. She infantilized them and destroyed them from the inside out so she could have steady supply. I remember Brian very young holding out his arms, saying, 'I love you Mommy,' and her slamming the door in his face." <<

seven

The Health Fallout
of Narcissistic Trauma

THE FUNDAMENTAL EXPERIENCE OF CHILDREN IN THE NARCISSISTIC HOME is not being seen. Lost inside themselves and incessantly preoccupied with their own restless neediness, narcissistic parents are effectively deaf, dumb, and blind. The child in the room is not a person busy with the work of forming her/his own complex selfhood, but rather a blank screen upon which such parents (one or both working in tandem) project their inner drama. When narcissistic parents look at their child, they merely see aspects of themselves. If the child is frightened by a stranger, these parents see their own fearful vulnerability, become ashamed and angry, and reject the child. If the child builds a tower, the parents see their own skillfulness, feel proud, and take ownership of the child.

As the child develops, s/he becomes less amenable to the parents' projected interpretations and must be manipulated into compliance. The rejected child must be continuously devalued to carry the parents' shame. And the owned (engulfed) child must be continuously idealized to carry their triumph. When the rejected child reacts against her/his role, the narcissistic parents see it as further evidence of that child's intransigence. When the owned child experiences success, again the parents see it as further evidence of their own worthiness. As long as both children perform their roles, there is a precarious balance. When the rejected child succeeds or the owned child fails, it is overlooked to maintain the balance. If the children diverge so much from their prescribed roles that it can no longer be ignored, narcissistic parents reassign the roles. Whichever role they play, the children are ciphers who remain unseen as long as their narcissistic parents define them. Their emotional negation is the essence of trauma and cannot be overstated. Trauma expert Bessel van der Kolk explains it this way:

> Trauma almost invariably involves not being seen, not being mirrored, and not being taken into account. . . . Being able to feel safe [and seen] with other people is probably the single most important aspect of mental health.[1]

CPTSD IN NARCISSISTICALLY ABUSED CHILDREN

Under siege, such children suffer the effects of long-term assaults to their sense of self that register in the body in devastating ways. These survivors are the walking wounded, emotionally and physically traumatized and at risk of further trauma. They become hypervigilant to attack, whether emotional, psychological, physical, or sexual, and their body's emergency response system (limbic system) is constantly activated, a state of hyperalert it is not designed for. Dr. van der Kolk describes the body's response to trauma:

> Ideally our stress hormone system should provide a lightning-fast response to threat, but then quickly return us to equilibrium. In PTSD [post-traumatic stress disorder] patients, however, the stress hormone system fails at this balancing act. Flight/fight/freeze signals continue after the danger is over. . . . Instead, the continued secretion of stress hormones is expressed as agitation and panic and, in the long term, wreaks havoc with their health.[2]

An aggregate of symptoms that result from traumatic experience, PTSD is often associated with veterans of war. But anyone who has endured distressingly devaluing, violent, life-threatening, or otherwise harmful circumstances or events may be left with emotional and physical manifestations of trauma that can persist for years. As opposed to PTSD, which arises from a single traumatic incident, complex post-traumatic stress disorder (CPTSD), a concept developed by psychiatrist Judith Herman, is the result of prolonged, repeated trauma[3] and encompasses a wider spectrum of possible symptoms. Children from narcissistic families typically develop symptoms of CPTSD that can continue and even worsen in adulthood unless addressed.[4] Symptoms vary but may include:

1. Hypervigilance
2. Feelings of helplessness
3. Difficulty regulating emotions
4. Insomnia
5. Nightmares
6. Flashbacks
7. Anxiety and panic attacks
8. Dissociation
9. Blank areas in memory
10. Avoidant behavior and procrastination
11. Phobias
12. Difficulty trusting others
13. Depression
14. Addictions
15. Anger
16. Hyperdefensiveness
17. Feelings of hopelessness
18. Search for rescuers/saviors
19. Search for mother or father figures
20. Social withdrawal and isolation
21. Risky or self-destructive behavior
22. A foreshortened sense of the future
23. Perfectionism
24. Defeatism and self-sabotage
25. A harsh inner critic
26. Devaluing self-talk
27. Disrupted breathing
28. Generalized guilt
29. Overcompliance or generalized defiance with authority
30. Compulsive self-effacement
31. A compromised immune system
32. A range of health problems, often mystifying to medical doctors

One of the most debilitating of these conditions is chronic sleep disturbance, which can include difficulty falling asleep, heightened sensitivity to
noise during sleep, and frequent awakenings,[5] as well as night terrors and
nightmares that may recur for decades. Such symptoms reflect disruptions
to the body's nervous system that worsen over time as a result of vicious cycles of sleep deprivation, anxiety about sleep, lowered immunity, and compromised health.

Washington, DC–based trauma and addiction specialist Regina Collins
described the narcissistic family as one where "everyone is rotating around
the narcissist on continual high alert, with consistently elevated stress levels
taking a heavy physical toll."[6] She compared the environment in the body
to driving a car with your feet simultaneously pressing hard on both the
accelerator and the brake. She explained how the resulting physiological
dysregulation can lead to addictive behavior that becomes a way of life in
adulthood:

> The sufferer seeks balance through behaviors that can become self-
> destructive but are meant to self-soothe: substance use, self-harm, obsessive
> gaming, gambling, and compulsive shopping. They give the brain a shot of
> dopamine for relief. It makes perfect sense from a coping standpoint.[7]

The narcissistically abused adult child's hypervigilant state is also associated with degraded health. San Francisco–based psychotherapist Julie
Tenenberg, who exclusively treats survivors of narcissistic abuse, said that *all*
of her patients with a narcissistic parent have significant health problems.
"Growing up in a narcissistic home places stress on the body that threatens
our homeostasis—the hypothalamic/pituitary/adrenal (HPA) axis."[8] The
HPA axis regulates our stress response and many body processes, including
digestion, immunity, emotion, and energy storage and release. When we
experience the physical assault of prolonged hypervigilance and disruptions
to the stress hormone cortisol, those processes break down and may result
in chronic disorders, such as the following:

- autoimmune disorders,
- cardiovascular problems,
- irritable bowel,
- arthritis and other connective tissue disorders,

- hypo- or hyperthyroidism,
- leaky gut,
- spinal problems,
- back and neck pain,
- migraines, and
- depleted adrenals.

Tenenberg pointed out that her clients frequently present with conditions that Western medical doctors don't pick up or acknowledge, an experience that mirrors the invalidation they grew up with and can reactivate trauma. Often such people suffer for years or decades with debilitating "mystery" problems that go unexplained and untreated. They may find themselves on an odyssey-like search for answers from both mainstream and alternative doctors, specialists, therapists, healers, shamans, gurus, and anyone else offering potential relief. Sufferers may face the double bind of financial hardship resulting from paying for treatments not covered by insurance that may or may not help, as well as a diminished ability to work.

NO CONTACT CAN HELP

Jeanie grew up with a narcissistic mother and an enabling father with narcissistic traits. Her mother routinely criticized and ridiculed Jeanie, publicly humiliating her and overtly favoring her other children. "My mother would wake me up early every Saturday morning to clean the house while she cuddled and giggled in bed with my younger sister until noon," Jeanie recalled. Her mother also restricted Jeanie's clothing and hairstyle while giving free rein to her other children.

By the time Jeanie was 17, she was suffering from symptoms that would later be diagnosed as stemming from multiple sclerosis. She also developed intense anxiety, depression, high blood pressure, migraines, and undiagnosed digestive problems. She said, "I felt like a walking black void, worthless and destroyed."

When Jeanie was finally tested for MS in her late 30s, she said her brain scan "lit up like a Christmas tree" with lesions, indicating that she had had the disease for years. Six years after she cut off contact with her family of origin, with support from her husband and children, a follow-up brain scan showed a dramatic reduction in lesions. "My doctor was amazed. She'd never seen anything like it," said Jeanie. "I'm convinced my lesions decreased because of going no contact." ««

GROOMED TO BE A VICTIM

When she went to college, Melissa was surprised to find herself telling a friend that she hated her father. The friend asked whether her father had abused her, and Melissa replied, "He loved me too much."

Around this time, she began to have symptoms of CPTSD, including insomnia, panic attacks, flashbacks, and nightmares about her father. Buried memories of his brutally beating her older brother surfaced. "My father was always picking on him. He'd swat him on the head and beat him with a belt," she said. By the time her brother was 9 (and Melissa 2), he was using drugs and stealing. When he was placed in a high-security juvenile facility as a teenager, their father disowned him.

"That was the last straw for my mother. She had wanted to get out of the marriage for a long time, and she finally left, saying she would never abandon her son," explained Melissa. By then, Melissa was 12 and since both parents wanted full custody, she was given the choice by a judge which parent she wanted to live with. She desperately wanted to choose her mother, but she feared her father's angry reprisal and felt responsible for his happiness, so she chose joint custody, living half the year with each parent. "My father had always painted himself as the victim in every situation, and I was still young enough to believe him. He also had been disabled in an accident by then, so I felt sorry for him."

Melissa said that at that point in her relationship with her father, "things got creepy and weird." He would take her in his camper into remote areas for weeks at a time. "He would force me to kiss him on the lips in a soft sensual way, and if I wore a skirt or shorts he would touch me on my thighs." Sometimes she would wake in a panic in the night, curled in a fetal position backed against the wall, seeing her father tiptoeing out of her bedroom. She said she has searched her memory and still doesn't know whether any overt sexual abuse occurred.

As she got to be an older teen, her father began stalking her. "He would show up during school field trips, pretending it was a coincidence, but that seemed crazy, and it began to freak me out," Melissa said. When she started seeing boys, her father followed her around on her dates. During her months with her mother, he would show up and sit in his car looking at Melissa through her bedroom window. Her mother took out a restraining order against him, but he continued to show up, parked just far enough to be beyond the legal boundary line.

Melissa had long felt that her relationship with her father was unhealthy and disturbing, but it wasn't until she entered therapy in her early 30s that she began to name her experience. Her counselor identified her father's narcissism and her role as a so-called golden child and helped her recognize the ways he had violated her boundaries.

Although Melissa's father never hit her, he often raged at and lectured her about why he was right and she was wrong. She said she learned to be a self-critical perfectionist to avoid making mistakes, and she became hypervigilant and intensely guarded because he would find ways to use innocent things against her, also a classic narcissistic behavior. "My fear of my father led to me being a people pleaser and sacrificer to survive. In retrospect I see I was groomed to be a victim."

Melissa has struggled with unhealthy relationships and poor boundaries, a common problem among adult children of narcissists (ACoNs). It took time before she found a loving and supportive relationship, but once she did, she was still afraid of getting married. "I eventually realized that it was because I couldn't stand the idea of my father being at the wedding and seeing me in my wedding dress."

At that point, Melissa decided to go no contact from her father. She sent him a letter and an article about narcissistic covert incest. "That's when the scapegoating began," she said. "He went public with the family about me victimizing him and my mother brainwashing me against him, and he roped my grandparents into it. My grandfather wrote me a blaming letter, and my grandmother started calling." Melissa's panic attacks returned, and she chose not to read or listen to their messages. Instead she had her therapist and husband field their attempts at contact to make sure "nothing truly scary was happening."

Melissa wrote a final letter to her father, explaining that she needed more time to heal before seeing him again. Not long after getting married, she found out her father had died. About his death, she said, "I felt numbness, and sadness that we never got to reach a resolution. There was also a certain amount of relief that he wouldn't be stalking me. I didn't have to watch my back anymore."

Melissa said she is starting to be more open about her family history, as a way to heal and also help others. She recently shared a story she wrote about her father at a public reading event. "It's a shameful history and hard to admit. Listeners were very supportive," she said. "When I was coming to this understanding there was so little information. I think it is important to be more open."

As for having kids of her own, now at 35 Melissa feels ready. Like so many ACoNs, for a long time she worried she would continue her family legacy and harm her children with her tendencies to be controlling and perfectionist. "For the first time in my life, I feel like I'm not having PTSD," she said. "Now I'm happily married with an incredibly supportive husband who understands and helps me focus on the future and step out of old dysfunctions. It's a forever battle, something I have to be aware of all the time." ‹‹

PART 3

THE NARCISSISTIC FAMILY

Rules and Roles in the Narcissistic Family

IN SIMPLE TERMS, A NARCISSISTIC FAMILY IS ONE IN WHICH THE NEEDS OF the parents are the focus and the children are expected in various ways to meet those needs. The healthy family model is turned on its head to support the parents rather than foster the children's development. As in other kinds of dysfunctional families, there is abuse and corresponding denial of the abuse. There is also an impoverishment of empathy, disrespect for boundaries, shaming treatment, ongoing turbulence, and an insistence on rigid role-playing.[1]

Children in the narcissistic family may (or may not) receive adequate caregiving and secure enough attachment in infancy, but as they increasingly individuate and express their own personalities, the parents resent and suppress their children's emerging needs and view the children as a means to get their own needs met.

Stephanie Donaldson-Pressman and Robert M. Pressman, in their groundbreaking book for clinicians *The Narcissistic Family: Diagnosis and Treatment*, describe the dynamic this way:

Somewhere between infancy and adolescence, the parents lose the focus (if they ever had it) and stop seeing the child as a discrete individual with feelings and needs to be validated and met. The child becomes, instead, an extension of the parents. Normal emotional growth is seen as selfish or deficient, and this is what is mirrored to the child. For the child to get approval, she must meet a spoken or unspoken need of the parent; approval is contingent on the child meeting the parent system's needs.[2]

THE NARCISSISTIC FAMILY PROFILE

1. Repressed Needs

Children in narcissistic families learn to meet their parents' needs while burying their own. They learn that to survive they must constantly work to read their parents' emotions while masking or faking theirs. Such children typically grow up feeling depressed, isolated, distrustful, self-doubting, and dislocated from their emotions, with little idea why. They may regard their parents and childhood as normal or even idyllic, yet carry around feelings of fear, anger, and despair.[3]

2. Hidden Dysfunction

Narcissistic families often appear relatively functional on the surface. This is because the narcissistic personality aspires to perfection and typically works to present a well-polished image of success to the world. Parents may have decent or even high-status jobs and keep up appearances, with children's material needs met. But, like a shiny red apple with mealy rot inside, below the surface sheen the children's emotional needs are ignored, resented, perhaps even maligned. The parents are emotionally unavailable to the children, while expecting their children to cater to them.

3. "Perfect" Parents

A particularly bedeviling aspect of life in the narcissistic home is that parents may send the message, directly or indirectly, that they are *the best parents on Earth* and expect their kids to mirror that back to them. Parents may even describe themselves as great, wonderful, or perfect mothers or fathers and actively work at building that image within their social circles and community. Their kids quickly learn never to question them or complain, while also giving constant recognition and reinforcement for anything they get, even minimal parenting. Often such parents expect their children to conform to their narrative for the family by presenting well in ways they value, whether it be academically, socially, artistically, athletically, or otherwise.

4. Denial and Secrecy

Family denial and secrecy are necessary to keep the narcissistic system running. Children must deny their real feelings and unmet needs. Siblings must not discuss with each other the family tensions and problems. And the family as a whole must present appearances of normalcy to the world. Thus children from the narcissistic family oftentimes are given no choice but to say (if not believe) that everything at home is okay, even exceptionally happy! In reality, they endure uniquely insidious and devastating trauma—trauma that can take decades to unravel and heal from. Typically, the understanding comes slowly (if at all), and the healing does not begin until the survivor has established significant perspective and distance from the family-of-origin dynamics.

RULES OF ENGAGEMENT

To support the parents, narcissistic homes have unspoken rules of engagement that dictate interactions among family members:

1. The Narcissist Is Always Right

This is the first rule that governs everyone's behavior. Anything less than full acceptance of the dominant narcissist's inherent correctness about all things is treason.

2. There Must Be Someone to Blame for Problems

If something bad happens, from a lost job to a spilled glass of milk, someone must be blamed for it, and that person will never be the narcissist.

3. Vulnerability Is Dangerous

Whether you missed the joke, dropped your fork, or had a hard day, showing vulnerability opens you to attack.

4. Mistakes Are Shameful

Making a mistake, even a harmless one, is cause for humiliation and shaming treatment.

5. You Must Take Sides

Just as there is always blame and shame, there are always sides, and if you aren't on the narcissist's side, you are wrong and you will lose.

6. There Is Never Enough Love/Respect to Go Around

Renewable resources in healthy families, love and respect are limited to the narcissist and whoever else is deemed worthy, usually the golden child. Respect for one person means disrespect for another.

7. Feelings Are Wrong

The feelings that make us human, that help us connect, get our needs met, and protect us from harm, are selfish and must be repressed. There is only room for the narcissist's feelings, and everyone else must set theirs aside to validate and cater to them.

8. Only One Side of an Argument Is Valid

Only the narcissist's opinion is acceptable, and disagreement with it is not tolerated.

9. Appearances Are More Important Than Substance

Even if everyone is suffering, they must smile for the family photo.

10. No One Is Forgiven

Mistakes and weaknesses, even ones we apologize for, are cause for mockery and condemnation that may continue for years.

11. Rage Is Normalized

Everyone is expected to swallow and endure the narcissist's irrational, explosive, and often violent rage. This may be magnified by other forms of mental illness or addiction.

12. Self-Control Is Required

Only the narcissist has free rein to express feelings, have emotional reactions, and make demands. Everyone else, except perhaps the golden child, must line up, shut up, and follow orders or suffer the consequences.

13. There Must Be a Scapegoat

Just as there must be blame, someone must be sacrificed to bear the main burden of the narcissist's projected self-loathing and the family's frustration and unhappiness.

14. Denial Is Rampant

Denial of abusive incidents, the atmosphere of fear, the ongoing mistreatment of the scapegoat, and routine forms of neglect is required to uphold the narcissist's delusions and maintain the family dysfunction.

15. There Is No Safety

Although the scapegoat is targeted with the brunt of the family abuse, everyone is on hyperalert because no one is safe from blame and rage.

"ORDINARY PEOPLE": PORTRAIT OF A NARCISSISTIC FAMILY (SPOILER ALERT)

The 1980 Oscar-winning best picture *Ordinary People*,[4] based on the novel by Judith Guest, presents one of the most fully realized depictions of a narcissistic family shown on film. In a breakout performance, Mary Tyler Moore plays Beth Jarrett, a narcissistic woman ensconced in an upper-crusty community on Chicago's suburban North Shore. Beth keeps a perfectly appointed home, charms at parties, and travels extensively with her well-earning husband, Calvin, a loving father but deluded and enabling husband played by Donald Sutherland.

Beth is the perfect-on-the-outside/sick-on-the-inside wife and mother: competent, pretty, slim, clever, well dressed, friendly, and fun-loving to the world, while callous, manipulative, angry, withholding, and unforgiving at home. Had it not been for a devastating family tragedy, her pathology might have gone unconfronted by Calvin and their teenage son Conrad, played by Timothy Hutton, who won an Oscar for the role.

Where the film's storytelling begins, Conrad has just returned home from a four-month hospitalization after a suicide attempt, and he and his parents are trying to get back on track with a gaping loss in their midst. We learn through flashbacks that while sailing on Lake Michigan, Conrad and his older brother Buck, an outgoing star athlete, ran afoul of a storm, and their boat capsized, in part because of Buck's carelessness. Clinging to the boat in roiling waters, Buck succumbed to exhaustion and drowned, while Conrad survived.

Judd Hirsch plays a rumpled, compassionate, straight-talking psychiatrist to the troubled Conrad, who gradually wakes up to his survivor's guilt and his mother's incapacity to love him. Beth never visited Conrad in the hospital and makes it known that she regards his depression and attempted suicide as shameful family blemishes. She is threatened that he is in therapy, angrily telling Calvin that the family's affairs should be kept private. In flashback scenes she swoons over Buck's attentions, basking in the glow of her favored golden child like an enamored schoolgirl, a striking contrast to her aloof disregard for Conrad's anguish and her brittle unresponsiveness when he repeatedly tries to reach out to her.

Conrad shows obvious symptoms of complex post-traumatic stress disorder (CPTSD): hypervigilance, depression, anxiety, insomnia, nightmares, loss of appetite. His CPTSD is emotional fallout from the boating tragedy but also common among scapegoated children and likely a condition that was developing before his brother's death.

Beth's narcissism is on display throughout the film, from her subtle recoil from Conrad's physical presence, to her coolly clipped speech and thinly masked punishing manner, to her disturbingly inappropriate infatuation with Buck, to her sexual and psychological manipulations of Calvin, to her trapped paralysis when Conrad gives her a conciliatory hug.

When Conrad finally confronts his mother about not visiting him in the hospital, he shouts, "You would have visited Buck if he had been in the hospital," to which she spits back, "Buck would have never been in the hospital!" Beth's and Calvin's picture-perfect marriage unravels as he increasingly questions her treatment of their son and her refusal to discuss difficult family truths, typical narcissistic denial and stonewalling. Near the end of the film, during a golf trip that Beth persuades Calvin to take over the holidays without Conrad along, Beth picks a fight and bitterly expresses the narcissist's defining cynicism and lack of empathy, qualities she projects onto others:

Calvin: "Can't you see anything except in terms of how it affects you?!"

Beth: "No! I can't! And neither can you and neither can anybody else, only maybe I'm just a little more honest about it."

As Calvin finally recognizes his wife's tragic inability to love, Beth stands her ground on footing that will soon betray her, or, more to the point, collapse under her betrayal.

About Conrad, Calvin tells her, "All he wants is to know that you don't hate him."

"God!" Beth says. "How could I hate him? Mothers don't hate their sons!" «

FAMILY ROLES

Irish playwright George Bernard Shaw famously called the family "a tyranny ruled by its weakest member," and there is no better example of this than the narcissistic one. At the helm of the narcissistic family is the demanding and unstable narcissist, usually a parent. Because of her/his extreme neediness, selfishness, and grandiosity, the narcissist dominates and manipulates family members to support her/his delusion of perfection and entitlement. Partners, children, and other relatives struggle to survive and manage their own needs, which are relegated to second priority far below the narcissist's.

In her influential book *Another Chance: Hope and Health for the Alcoholic Family*, Sharon Wegscheider-Cruse first introduced the idea of common roles in the alcoholic family,[5] which quickly became the model for understanding roles in dysfunctional families more generally. The roles are addict, enabler/codependent, hero, scapegoat, mascot, and lost child. These roles emerge in the narcissistic family, with the narcissist as addict and the additional role of the golden child replacing or overlapping with the hero role, or the scapegoat overlapping with the hero role.

Narcissist

This is usually a parent or parents but may be a child/sibling. The narcissist is in essence the family tyrant whom everyone else revolves around, scrambling to cope as best they can. There also may be a hive of narcissists in grandparents and other relatives. As we have discussed, people with NPD lack a firm identity, resilient self-esteem, and emotional (as opposed to cognitive) empathy for others, making them excessively needy while also pathologically self-serving, reactive, and often cruel. They may express their narcissism in exhibitionist self-aggrandizing dominance or more closet passive-aggressive manipulations. They may be primarily selfish, blaming, and callous, or in more extreme cases, malicious and violent.

Two Narcissistic Parents

It is not uncommon for both parents in a narcissistic home to be at least somewhat narcissistic. Research shows that narcissists are more tolerant than most of narcissism in others, including in couple relationships and friendships. Psychologist Susan Krauss Whitbourne describes one study's findings this way:

> The upshot of the study is that it is not only possible for those high in narcissism to become and stay a couple, but that they do so. We tend to think of fulfilling long-term relationships as requiring a willingness to put the partner first, but for those unable to do so, this study's findings show that there are partners for even the seemingly least lovable.[6]

In such partnerships, one may play the openly combative role to the other's "nice," "reasonable," or long-suffering victim routine, or some variation on that theme. Or one parent is narcissistic and the other may be mentally/emotionally impaired in some other way, for example with anxiety, depression, or another form of personality disorder, such as borderline, obsessive-compulsive, or substance use disorder. Children in such dynamics may blame the more overtly difficult parent and deny the dysfunctional behavior of the other parent because seeing both as pathologically selfish or otherwise impaired presents an overwhelmingly threatening reality. Often such confusion and denial can persist well into adulthood, with adult children perhaps even idealizing the "good" parent as innocent victim, "saint," "nicest person you could ever meet," and so forth.

Enabling Closet Narcissist

In some cases, an enabler may be a closet narcissist impressed with the apparent confidence or outward success of a more exhibitionist narcissist.[7] Such an enabler may admire the other narcissist and feed her/his self-esteem and identity by living vicariously through that partner. Or the more closet narcissist may derive satisfaction and social attention and approval from managing the exhibitionist narcissist's difficult and selfish personality. In such a relationship, the narcissistic enabler may present her-/himself as the long-suffering good/kind/loyal/patient/reasonable victim who deserves better, while being selfish and exploitative below the surface. As parents, both narcissistic partners enable each other by overlooking and/or supporting their negligent and abusive behavior toward their children.

Enabler/Codependent Partner

Narcissists' primary enabler is typically their partner/spouse. They also may have enabling relatives, friends, employees, students, congregants, constituents, and the like. In some cases, the narcissist's main enabler is a favored child under the delusion that s/he is the only one who can manage that parent's happiness. Such children often construct their identity around the demands of the parent, constantly working to please and appease.

Enabling partners support the narcissist's precious persona and abusive behavior by unquestioningly accepting her/his version of reality, cleaning up her/his messes, and acting as an apologist for her/him while also absorbing much of her/his abuse. Enablers are often drawn in without understanding their situation as one that enables abuse. They may feel confused by the narcissist's brainwashing messages, constantly working to avoid conflict and manage the chaos. Enablers are commonly under the delusion that they are the only one who can truly understand the narcissist and meet her/his needs. Enablers make abuse possible by sustaining the dysfunctional status quo. Moreover, enablers allow the narcissist to avoid the consequences of her/his actions and prevent the family from potentially overcoming its unhealthy patterns.

People who partner with a narcissist often come from a narcissistic or otherwise dysfunctional background where they learned codependent patterns of behavior (see Chapter 13). Codependent people tend to have low self-esteem, neglect their own needs, define themselves heavily in relation to their partner, and are addicted to feeling needed. They often have pre-existing psychological and physical addictions to abuse cycles and see such relationship dynamics as inevitable or normal.[8]

Narcissistic Grandparents

Since narcissism tends to pay it forward generationally, where there are narcissistic parents, there are often narcissistic grandparents, as well as aunts, uncles, and/or cousins. And don't forget the in-laws! As grandparents, narcissists seldom behave better than they did as parents, and they are likely to try to leverage whatever power they may have, such as financial support or social influence, to continue to dominate the family. If given the chance, they may assign roles, in particular, favorites and scapegoats, to their grand-children as they did with their kids. Since they have less control once their children are adults, they may rely primarily on indirect forms of manipulation, such as triangulating (see Chapter 9).

When adult children of narcissists have kids of their own, there can be a major shift in how they see their family of origin. Such parents may only have a nascent understanding of what they grew up with and may still be blaming themselves for how they were treated, so it often comes as a shock to find their children receiving similar treatment. This may push adult children of narcissists to reassess the family dynamics and establish healthier boundaries to protect their kids.

 CENTER STAGE

Sawyer's father always needed to be center stage, and the rest of the family had learned not to compete with him. Then, Sawyer's outgoing son came along. "My son is confident, and this does not play well around his grandfather. Recently, at his sixth birthday party, he was excited to pick the first slice of pizza, but Dad grabbed one before he could, and gloated while he ate it. My son took it well. When the cake came around, he snapped up a slice before his grandfather got there, and everyone had a laugh. Everyone except Dad, who left the party in an angry huff," Sawyer said. «

Scapegoat

Narcissistic parents project their shame and self-hatred on the scapegoat. As the sacrificial goat of the family, the scapegoat carries the blame for family misfortunes and, in doing so, allows it to avoid looking at its core problems. Such a child may be the "disloyal" truth teller who stands up to the narcissist and questions the family system or the "angry" rebel who acts out at home and possibly gets in trouble at school.

Sibling attitudes toward a targeted child can range from fully participating in the scapegoat's abuse, to passively sympathizing with the scapegoat, to attempting to defend him or her. If the scapegoat excels or the golden child disappoints, parents sometimes elevate the scapegoat to the golden child role, a status s/he may embrace, accept with ambivalence, or outright reject depending on how much perspective s/he has about the family dysfunction.

As a result of the ongoing blame foisted on scapegoats, they often carry intense shame, self-doubt, and self-destructive tendencies that can hobble them in adulthood. Their long-term trauma can cause debilitating CPTSD and lead to ongoing health and financial problems, creating a vicious cycle that further exacerbates their suffering. Family members may feel varying levels of concern or bewilderment about the scapegoat's struggles or regard such problems as further justification of his or her outcast role.

But while scapegoats may be dogged by difficulties, they are also most likely to break out of the family dysfunction. Their outsider status, combined with an inner strength and independent-mindedness that may have put them at odds with their narcissistic parents in the first place, can motivate them to confront the family dynamics and seek greater understanding and healing as adults. Often highly empathetic in response to being bullied and because they were trained to consider others' need before their own, they have the potential to transcend narcissistic patterns and forge meaningful connections in and beyond the family. Their biggest challenge is to recognize their own codependent patterns and replace them with self-care and self-respect. See Chapters 15 and 17 for more about the scapegoat role.

 MOCKINGBIRD

Carla's father baited her on a regular basis. One day when she was 12, she was standing holding a glass of milk while her father yelled at her. "I acted calm, but my blood was boiling," she said. He began egging her on to throw the milk. "Come on, do it! You're angry! You know you want to throw that glass," he goaded. "Go ahead. You're furious. Throw it, throw it!" Carla finally threw the glass. "Then for a while, it became a kind of game," she recalled. Her father would tell her what an angry person she was and bait her to throw things. "I started throwing plates like Frisbees. It was crazy." After Carla gave in to her father's provocations, he would laugh with triumph. "It felt awful, and after a while I realized it was wrong, so I stopped," she said. But her father never let her forget. "It never ended, for years, hearing those stories of what an awful angry kid I was." ‹‹

Flying Monkeys

Often one or more children/adult children or other relatives in the narcissistic family, flying monkeys are enablers who also perpetrate the narcissist's abuse on targeted victims. Like the flying monkeys in *The Wizard of Oz*, they accept the narcissist's alternative reality, assist in the narcissist's cruelties and smear campaigns, and carry out abuse by proxy.

There is a fine line between enabling and acting as a flying monkey. Often, enablers cross that line to avoid being targeted themselves or because they are invested in believing the lies that justify the narcissist's abuse of others, particularly scapegoated children. For scapegoats, the betrayal of the enabling codependent parent may be harder to accept and forgive than that of the narcissist because they view the enabler as the "safe" parent who should know better. Flying monkeys may be narcissistic themselves.

Narcissists typically also have people outside the family, such as friends, employees, neighbors, and other community members, who act as flying monkeys. Unaware, naive, sycophantic, or narcissistic themselves, they become involved in the narcissist's dramas and unknowingly or knowingly assist in harming selected victims. For recipients of such treatment, particularly children, the experience can be devastating.

Golden Child

The golden child is the family favorite, on whom special attention, praise, and privilege are bestowed. Narcissists project what they want to believe about themselves onto their idealized offspring and engulf the child's identity into their own. Children put in this role are typically pressured to excel and fulfill outward appearances of success for the family. They also may be spoiled, infantilized, and/or shielded from the harsh treatment others get.

Favored children experience a complex mixture of emotions. They may feel confusion and guilt about the favoritism they receive compared with the unwarranted abuse of other family members. They are likely to feel burdened with a sense of responsibility to manage and appease the narcissistic parent while being afraid that parent will turn on them or hurt their other parent or siblings. They may love and admire sisters and brothers and feel rejected and isolated because their siblings have withdrawn from them. Or they may internalize the family values and adopt their parent's narcissism, including hostility toward the scapegoat.

The privileged status of favored children can make them smug and superior but also insecure about their real worth outside the family. As objects of idealized attention, they may struggle with confusing dualities of arrogance and guilt, perfectionism and self-sabotage, exaggerated power and helplessness, and an underlying impostor syndrome. They often have trouble individuating from the dominant narcissistic parent and, in adulthood, establishing authentic identities of their own and intimacy with others. Sometimes golden children come out of denial and confront the family dysfunction if they become scapegoated by their parents or if their partner and/or children are scapegoated. A willingness to acknowledge and separate from the family dysfunction is crucial for the golden child to break the cycle and form balanced and fulfilling relationships in adulthood. See Chapters 15 and 17 for more about the golden child role.

BOY'S BOY

Nate was the family golden child who got in trouble at school but was excused by his father, who said he was just a spirited "boy's boy." At home, Nate had always picked on his scapegoated little brother William, with whom he shared a bedroom. When Nate was 12 and William 7, Nate began masturbating in front of him, and soon he was holding his little brother down and raping him. He would beat William in places under his clothes where people wouldn't see. Sometimes the boys' parents noticed William's bruises and said he was clumsy. William begged his mother to let him sleep with her, but his father would become infuriated and send him away, saying he was a "mama's boy." When William finally told his parents about Nate's sexual abuse, his father excused his brother and called it "normal curiosity." «

Hero/Caretaker

Often the oldest child, the family hero assumes a problem-solving, caretaking, and/or high-achieving role. The hero responds to the family turbulence by trying to instill order and excelling in certain areas, such as academics or sports, that bring pride to the family. Family heroes tend to be hypercapable, doing well in school and perhaps taking on responsibilities that would normally be filled by a parent, such as cleaning, cooking, caring for siblings, or earning money. They may build their identity around "saving" their family or defending a scapegoated parent or siblings from overt abuse.

Heroes who confront the family dysfunction may be perceived as a threat and become targeted as scapegoats. Family heroes also may be cast aside if they fail to fulfill family expectations or if a different child or a parent's new romantic partner steps into the role. When a hero child is replaced by a new adult, as when a parent remarries, that child may feel intense betrayal and abandonment.

Heroes typically experience ambivalence about their role, feeling needed and special but also burdened and trapped. They may feel confused about their own agency, feeling at once powerful in their capabilities but also helpless to ultimately change the underlying family dysfunction and get their needs met. As adults, they are often drawn into further caretaking or justice-seeking roles and struggle with control issues and feelings of perfectionism and overresponsibility. They typically carry the unconscious belief that they can only receive love by earning it. Finding a balance between giving and receiving in their relationships and work lives is often the biggest challenge for hero children. As with other family members, self-awareness and reexamining family dynamics is important for personal growth and healing. Shedding the compulsive desire to rescue or fix other people and learning to accept support is the path to well-being and healthier relationships. See Chapters 15 and 17 for more about the hero/caretaker role.

Lost Child

Children in the role of lost child adapt to the family stress by keeping a low profile, making few demands, and avoiding conflict. They disappear into themselves, attracting neither negative nor positive attention. They are often quiet, separating from family drama by drifting into fantasy and disconnecting from their feelings. They typically stay out of trouble and do well enough in school to coast along, allowing family members to point to them as evidence of the family's normalcy.

In reality, lost children are victims of neglect and emotional abuse. Their withdrawal helps buffer them from the family chaos, but it comes at great personal cost. As adults, they are likely to struggle to communicate and understand their emotions. Relationships are difficult for them, as they tend to dismiss or deny their feelings, disown their needs, and socially isolate. If they can overcome their tendency to self-efface and resist intimacy, they can find healing by building self-awareness, connecting with others, and expressing themselves creatively. See Chapters 15 and 17 for more about the lost child role.

Mascot

The family mascot learns early on to receive attention and diffuse tensions by performing. Often the youngest and/or "cute" child, the mascot plays the role of court jester who uses humor and entertainment to distract family members from unhappiness and conflict. Mascots may reveal family truths through wisecracking while appeasing with comedic relief. Like the golden child, they are often treated with favoritism and excused from responsibility and blame.

Mascots are easily distracted and may have trouble staying on task at school or work. As adults, mascot personalities can take longer than most to mature, struggle to understand their emotions, and fall into excessive people-pleasing. They are often anxious and fearful, feelings they try to out-run with frenetic social lives and possible addictions. Resisting the urge to distract and overextend themselves socially and dedicating more time to self-reflection, self-care, and rewarding work are roads to healing. See Chapters 15 and 17 for more about the mascot role.

Narcissistic Child

In some instances, the primary narcissist in a family is a child/adult child. Although most people who develop NPD come out of families with at least one narcissistic parent, other circumstances can give rise to pathological narcissism in a child. Parents may be extremely rigid and/or permissive, or there may be traumatizing conditions, owing to death, substance abuse, religious extremism, or mental illness other than narcissism in the family. Parents who grew up in a narcissistic family who did not develop pathological narcissism themselves may nevertheless model narcissistic behaviors and values to their own children that result in NPD. Such parents suffered narcissistic abuse in their family of origin and find themselves facing it again in their own child, a familiar but acutely distressing reality. For parents with emotional intelligence and empathy, managing such a child is a lifelong struggle and source of profound sorrow. These parents may find themselves caught in cycles of anxiety, guilt, anger, and helplessness, which may be exacerbated by destructive interference from narcissistic parents/grandparents and other relatives.

Recognizing the problem early in the child's life and actively working to support that child's development of resilient self-esteem, self-awareness, self-control, and empathy for others can help replace narcissistic patterns with healthier ways of being in the world. However, reaching the point of identifying a child's narcissism and need for intervention usually requires a willingness in the parents to confront the dysfunction in their own families of origin, personalities, and parenting styles. Sadly, parents unwilling to do such work often seal the fates of their children and perpetuate the generational trauma.

Narcissistic Sibling

Similarly, for more emotionally stable siblings, life with a narcissistic brother or sister can seem like a minefield of exploitation, reactivity, outsize demands, and possibly betrayal and outright abuse. It may feel like everything revolves around the narcissistic sibling, with that child gobbling up attention and all too frequently being excused from outrageous behavior. Children under such conditions may feel pressure to balance the selfishness of their narcissist sibling by being self-effacing, hyperresponsible, and/or hypersensitive superkids. They are likely to repress their own needs and rightful anger and may go to great lengths to understand and excuse their antagonistic sibling for the sake of peace in the family.

Because children are keenly attuned to issues of fairness, especially in relation to siblings, the innately unjust nature of life with a narcissistic personality is a painful reality to bear. The neurotypical child's suffering is further magnified when parents are in denial about the narcissistic child's problems and perhaps functioning as codependent enablers of that child's abusive behavior. Children with a narcissistic sibling also face the confusion and pain of rarely or never feeling their love and loyalty reciprocated by that sibling. Such children, particularly younger ones, are naturally bewildered by their sister's or brother's competitive and callous treatment, and they may work for years to get attention, approval, and affection that never come. The best way to help children in this position is to acknowledge reality, including the narcissistic sibling's limitations; teach them that they are not responsible for how their sibling acts or treats them; protect them from potential abuse; and give them ways to gain independence from the family drama.

Fluid and Changing Roles

Identifying patterns in the narcissistic family can be very helpful, but it is important to understand that rules and roles are fluid and changeable, and children may serve different functions from day to day and when family dynamics change or a sibling leaves home. A child also may play a different primary role with each parent, particularly if parents are separated or divorced. For example, a child who is frequently scapegoated in one parent's home may function as a hero/caretaker in his or her other parent's home. Similarly, roles can overlap, such as when a child functions as a mascot/golden child or scapegoat/lost child. In single-child families, the child may take on aspects of some or all of the different roles, depending on the moment.

Regardless of roles, for everyone in the narcissistic family the defining experience is tension, instability, and insufficient adult support. Children, even favored ones, inevitably experience hypercriticism, unrealistic expectations, and neglect of their need for nurturance and secure individuation. They cannot help but strain under the weight of the narcissistic parents' incessant, pathological delusions and demands.

    A HERO-SCAPEGOAT'S STORY

Jason's father, Gregory, was an exhibitionist narcissist and high-functioning alcoholic who overcompensated for his insecurities with arrogance, self-aggrandizement, and competitive one-upmanship. He frequently flew into rages, breaking things, kicking and punching walls and furniture, blasting music, and driving recklessly. He routinely mocked his family and friends in the guise of humorous teasing, pointing out embarrassing mistakes and flaws and laughing uproariously at his own cruel jokes. A successful businessman, Gregory was clever and at times funny and engaging, and he used those qualities to attract—and exploit—family, friends, customers, and employees.

Gregory treated his cherished daughter, Susan, as the family golden child, engulfing her as a can-do-no-wrong extension of himself. He assigned the role of family scapegoat to his son, Jason. As the oldest child in the family, Jason served as a target of blame for his sister's frequent forgetfulness and for Gregory's projections of self-hatred, receiving the brunt of his ridicule and rage.

When Jason questioned or disagreed with his father, Gregory regularly verbally attacked him and projected his aggression by claiming that Jason was angry and unfair to his perfect dad. Gregory denigrated Jason's interest in music and indifference to sports, and he often praised Susan's good looks, logical mind, and athleticism. Although Susan loved her brother, she did not defend Jason or question her father's behavior, partly for fear of losing her status and becoming targeted herself. Her father's anger frightened her, but she worked hard not to show it and refused to discuss it when Jason tried to talk about it with her, calling him too sensitive as her father did.

Jason's younger stepbrothers functioned as the family's lost child and mascot. The older of the two, Brett, was quiet. He liked drawing and reading science fiction and spent most of his time in his room. He did fine in school but was never a standout, and he didn't argue or cause trouble. When Gregory picked on him at the dinner table, Jason would defend Brett, sometimes coming to verbal blows with his father. The youngest, Blake, was likable and outgoing, and he made the family laugh with outlandish stories. He was popular at school and by third grade had a full social calendar and was staying most nights at friends' houses. Jason worried about Blake being gone so much and tried to look out for him.

Jason's stepmother, Penny, enabled Gregory by enduring his abuse, failing to protect her sons from his attacks, and abetting the maintenance of Susan's role as golden child and Jason's as scapegoat. Although Penny and Susan resented each other, Penny never questioned Susan's princesslike status and often used Jason as a deflective target to avoid Gregory's line of fire on herself and her sons. She helped Gregory maintain his dominance over the family by blaming Jason arbitrarily and going along with Gregory's insistence that Jason was an angry troublemaker. Although Jason was aware that his father had problems, and at times challenged the family dynamics, he also internalized blame and sought love and approval that was alternately withheld or offered like a carrot to feed his father's need for control and attention.

Things were different for Jason and Susan when they stayed with their mother, Margot. Before their parents divorced, Jason often tried to protect his mother from Gregory's outbursts. After they split up, Margot struggled with depression and Jason stepped up to handle responsibilities around the house. She talked a lot about the breakup, and Jason listened, reassuring her that she was a good person, attractive, and capable. Jason had never spent so much time with his mother, who had usually focused on Gregory, and he felt proud to be helping her. He stopped hanging out with his friends so she wouldn't be alone after school while Susan was at swim practice. When Margot got involved with a serious boyfriend, she abruptly shifted her attention away from Jason, who felt like he had lost his best friend.

Susan was a talented swimmer who seemed self-assured but struggled with an eating disorder that she hid from Gregory. She became arrogant and competitive as an adult and went into business like her father, while Jason took an unconventional path as a musician. Jason pursued therapy and came to understand that he had played scapegoat with his father and hero/caretaker with his mother. He recognized his dependence on pills as a symptom of post-traumatic stress. When he became a father, he quit drugs and shielded his own children from his family's dysfunction with firm boundaries and limited contact. In contrast, Susan was openly critical of her own son as her father had been of Jason. Since she did not shield him from Gregory's attacks, her son filled the role of the new family scapegoat. <<

nine

Patterns in the Narcissistic Family

JUST AS THERE ARE COMMON ROLES IN NARCISSISTIC FAMILIES, THERE ARE also patterns that characterize life in such homes: isolation, rage, projection, shaming, gaslighting, triangulating, cognitive distortions, smear campaigns, and tragedy, such as suicide.

ISOLATION

One of the most insidious and debilitating aspects of life in a narcissistic home is isolation. Family members are cut off from support because very few people truly understand narcissism. This is compounded by the fact that narcissists actively work to alienate their partners and children from the outside world, from one another, and from their own sense of reality.

Narcissists Isolate Family Members from People Outside the Family

The thinking and behavior patterns of people with NPD are so far outside of normal rules of engagement that they are virtually impossible to comprehend unless you've lived with them (or something like them, such as addiction) firsthand. Most people, even if they know something about the disorder, have no idea what narcissistic abuse really entails, and they are unaware of its profound and lasting damage. As a survivor, even once you are away from the narcissist, you struggle to understand what you have been through. Essentially you have been abused and at the same time gaslighted into believing it never happened or was your fault (or the fault of some other abused member of your family). Moreover, the narcissists have likely told you in a thousand ways that you (or another abused family member) have actually wronged *them*. Tragically, when survivors reach out for support, their friends, relatives, pastors, and even therapists out of ignorance may minimize or dismiss their experience, further undermining and isolating them. Such people, unaware of narcissistic family dynamics, may give dangerous advice to survivors, such as to confront or reconcile with an abusive spouse or parent.

Isolation from the world beyond the family also occurs because narcissists typically prefer to keep family members cut off as a way to control and weaken them. They keep careful watch over what family information is shown to others and discourage relationships with people they view as a threat to their mask. They will also undermine supportive relationships their family members may have with relatives, friends, teachers, coaches, and the like, as a way to keep them more dependent and compliant.[1] For the same reason, narcissists also may encourage certain relationships their children and partner may have that they see as advantageous to them in some way.

Narcissists Isolate Family Members from One Another

Another common behavior, conscious and unconscious, of narcissists is to divide and conquer within the family. One method they use is to treat children inequitably, favoring some and targeting others. They also create a competitive and threatening atmosphere that keeps family members vying for approval and/or reprieve from attack. Attack can take many forms, including rage, ridicule, and blame. Narcissists typically isolate their partners with a host of abuse, from criticism to violent outbursts, guilt to silent treatment. Partners often compound children's isolation by supporting divisions within the family. Or they may further isolate themselves by absorbing the narcissist's abuse to protect their children.

Narcissists Isolate You from Yourself

In addition to weakening connections you have both outside and inside the family, narcissists undermine your self-confidence and connection to reality. They gaslight family members by routinely questioning or denying their perceptions and projecting their own abuse and corrupt reasoning onto them. This creates a cognitive dissonance, or conflict between what you perceive to be true and what the narcissist tells you is happening, that breeds confusion and self-doubt and makes you more susceptible to manipulation.

RAGE

Rage plays an ever-present and brutalizing role in the narcissistic family. Whether it is overtly displayed with yelling and violence or sublimated in passive-aggressive form through silent treatment, stonewalling, blame, sarcasm, or guilt, rage drives the narcissist and shapes life in a narcissistic home.

Most people driven to anger begin gradually with emotions of stress and annoyance that progress into a more heated confrontational state. Emotionally healthy people give warning signs that they are frustrated, and they attempt to communicate before their feelings develop into full-on anger. Those familiar with narcissistic rage, on the other hand, know that it is usually right at the surface and ready to blow at light speed. Exhibitionist narcissists in particular often skip normal stages of anger and in a half-breath leap to rage as flattening as a tornado and often involving some kind of physical violence. Even when a narcissist is apparently calm, family members remain on guard for possible sudden attack.

Adding to the trauma, narcissists rarely apologize for or even acknowledge their rage. Instead they often project their own irrational attacking behavior onto others they have traumatized, typically a scapegoated child or partner, further increasing the abused person's distress. In narcissists' eyes, they are always the victim, never the victimizer, and their behavior is always justified because they must see themselves as perfect and above reproach.

There is no easy way to deal with narcissists' rage, but it helps to understand its source and realize that it is not personal even when narcissists say it is. Narcissists operate with a terrible hypervigilance that they, ironically, also engender in others. Their sense of emotional vulnerability is so intense and their overcompensating grandiosity so extreme that they are always defending against perceived snubs and humiliations, which they continuously interpret around them as real experience. Day-to-day lows or minor rejections that all of us endure are magnified for narcissists as shattering seismic disturbances. Life's smallest slights, such as being kept waiting or given perfunctory service, can trip narcissists' alarm system, leading to fury and vengeful reactions.

People within a narcissist's sphere quickly acquire their own detection system for reading the narcissist's moods and avoiding anything that might trigger her/his rage. Family members in particular become hypervigilant, learning how to placate the narcissist and, if possible, prevent confrontation and conflagration. As we have discussed, hypervigilance and avoidance, along with a range of other debilitating emotions, especially in developing children, cause emotional and physiological problems that can last a lifetime.

One of your biggest challenges in dealing with narcissistic rage, as difficult as enduring the narcissist's emotional and often physical violence, is unlearning the habit of blaming yourself for it—something the person with NPD constantly manipulates others to do. The narcissist's mantras are "It's your fault" and "You made me do it." Whether you are the child, adult child, partner/spouse, or even another family member, friend, coworker, or employee of a narcissistically disordered individual, you are likely to doubt yourself and take responsibility for things the narcissist does that are not only not your fault but, in fact, hurt you.

Whatever harm the narcissist does, if you are her/his primary scapegoat s/he finds a reason—however convoluted—to hold you responsible. Particularly if you have a narcissistic parent, perhaps your most important lesson is to understand that the narcissist's disorder, unhappiness, and rage are not your responsibility. Repeat: *The narcissist's problems are not your fault and not your responsibility.*

BREATHING AGAIN

Mimi's father beat her throughout her childhood. She has no idea how many times her nose was broken, but it wasn't until her mid-40s, after extensive reconstructive surgery, that she recalled breathing normally. "The surgeon had to build a whole new nose from scratch because my septum and valves were collapsed," Mimi explained. "It was the most amazing thing. I had never breathed through my nose in my memory." ≪

PROJECTION

Psychological projection in simple terms is the act of attributing uncomfortable (negative or positive) feelings or qualities in oneself to others. We all project from time to time, because it can be easier to have other people "carry" certain emotions than to acknowledge them in ourselves. Our emotions can feel threatening any time they contradict how we see or wish to see ourselves or how we think others wish to see us.

On a fundamental level, all narcissists' relationships are exercises in negative or positive projection, and projection dominates relationships and interactions in the narcissistic family. Narcissists treat their children and spouse as projection screens for their intolerable shame and vulnerability and their grandiose fantasies. They also project their abusive behavior to deflect blame and responsibility and to control family members. As a result, spouses and children struggle with cognitive dissonance and distorted beliefs about themselves and others.

Negative Projection

Lacking the emotional resources to acknowledge and process their feelings of shame and continuously being overwhelmed by them, narcissists attempt to exorcise their shame by projecting it outward onto others. Anything they feel ashamed about is likely to become someone else's problem.

Negative narcissistic projection serves several purposes. It allows narcissists to:

1. Displace painful emotions
2. Make someone else carry their intolerable feelings
3. Divert negative attention away from themselves
4. Avoid responsibility and blame
5. Feel and look good in comparison with someone else

In general, projection is more convincing, both to others and oneself, if it touches on a degree of truth about the recipient. Harping on a child's childishness, for example, is harder to argue with because children *are* childish by virtue of the fact that they are children. But often with narcissistic projection, the very thing narcissists are finding fault with in the person they are projecting onto not only is the narcissists' issue but is also *created* by the narcissists. For instance, a narcissistic parent accuses her teenaged son of being an angry person because he reacts with anger to her frequent rage and verbal attacks. His anger about her habitual assault is justified, but she reframes the situation to place accountability on him, displacing responsibility and blaming the victim.

Blaming the Victim

Blaming the victim is a form of projection that is as old as the hills. It is an effective strategy for further disarming those under attack by leveraging their vulnerability. Victim blaming gains traction in families and society at large because it enables us to ignore disturbing evidence before us that the world can be a brutal, unsafe, and unjust place. Studies dating back to the 1960s show that humans are in fact predisposed to defend their need to believe in a just world by projecting blame onto victims of violence or misfortune. We blame rape victims, for example, when we accuse them of provoking the perpetrator, and poor people when we accuse them of laziness, poor judgment, or stupidity.[2]

Narcissists compulsively blame to shift their sense of shame, and they victim-blame their own abusive behavior to deflect responsibility and further weaken the target's defenses by

- creating confusion and self-doubt in the target,
- leading the target to blame him- or herself, and
- undermining the target's credibility with others.

Blaming the victim is a form of scapegoating that plays out in some form in nearly all narcissistic families. Family members typically participate in victim-blaming because it is easier to believe that the family scapegoat deserves the treatment s/he receives than that the universe of home is an unjust place where cruelties and inequities are the norm. Enablers often subscribe to scapegoating to avoid being targeted themselves, and they justify their role in the scapegoating through victim-blaming. Anyone, including a partner, child, adult child, or even a pet, may be scapegoated. For scapegoats, victim-blaming adds further trauma to their experience of abuse. They are attacked, disbelieved, and held responsible for the pain inflicted upon them, while the narcissist and those acting as flying monkeys are fortified in their tribalistic gang mentality.

BLAME THE VICTIM

Christine's grandfather began raping her when she was 11 years old. Her parents were often out for the night, leaving her under her grandfather's supervision. He told her she was a "bad girl," that what he did was her fault, and that her parents would hate and disown her if she said anything about what she "made him do." In time, Christine grew withdrawn and angry. Her grades dropped, and she avoided being home by spending time on the streets with other kids. Finally, during a fight with her mother, she said her grandfather had been forcing her to have sex. When her mother told Christine's father, he accused Christine of seducing her grandfather and ruining the family. He kicked her out of the house, leaving her homeless at 15. <<

Positive Projection

Projection can involve "positive" emotions and traits as well as negative ones. People doing the projecting may ascribe to someone else desirable qualities that they are uncomfortable about within themselves or feel are deficient in themselves.[3] Idealization is a form of positive projection that happens when we fall in love. In our idealized partner, we may see parts of ourselves we value but have been taught to disown, or we may see nascent things we wish to develop in ourselves, viewing the object of our idealization as a means to complete ourselves.

Idealization in love is normal, but in longer-term relationships both people involved must be able to transition into a more realistic view of each other to sustain a healthy connection. To allow for genuine intimacy and growth in the relationship and to avoid disappointment, the objectified mate must be allowed to become a fully realized and therefore also flawed person—a subject rather than an object. Similarly, children tend to idealize their parents but gradually come to see them more realistically over time as they grow up. A more mature understanding of our parents helps us develop a resilient acceptance of ourselves and our loved ones as we age.

The Shifting Ground of Idealization and Devaluation

People with NPD frequently idealize others and lack the ability to sustain realistic relationships. Because they vacillate internally between feelings of defectiveness and entitled superiority, they also simplistically categorize others as worthless or wonderful. Demanding perfection in themselves, they demand it in those around them, which inevitably gives way to destructive disillusionment. Typically their mates and children, siblings and friends are treated to continuous reappraisal, a roller-coaster ride of idealization and devaluation, if not abandonment. Even an idealized golden child is rarely spared devaluation. The narcissistic parent's binary thinking, shifting agenda, lack of loyalty, and harsh assessment of others mean s/he will perceive fatal flaws in everyone eventually. In narcissists' irrational and ruthless family hierarchy, golden children may lose their privileged status, and scapegoated children may be invited to wear the golden crown. The only way to truly avoid narcissists' insistence on hierarchical roleplaying is to disengage from the family drama.

 ## THE BEST OF TIMES AND THE WORST OF TIMES

Haley lived with her mother and spent summers with her father. As summer grew closer, he would call and text her, talking about how much fun they would have and the amazing things they would do together. Things were great for the first few weeks of her visits but quickly disintegrated as her father grew impatient, critical, and eventually verbally abusive and withdrawn. Often, Haley would call her mother and ask to come home early. "I wouldn't hear from him for months afterward," she said. "Then at some point after Christmas, he'd start contacting me again, and the cycle would repeat." It wasn't until Haley found a coach who understood narcissistic abuse that she came to recognize her father's fluctuating pattern of idealization and disappointment about their time together. "I felt it was my fault, like I was always ruining things. It took me a long time to stop blaming myself," she said. ‹‹

SHAMING

Often confused with its cousin *guilt*, which is a feeling of distress about something we have done, *shame* is a feeling of distress about who we are. Simply put, guilt is "I *did* something bad," whereas shame is "I *am* bad." Narcissists rarely feel guilt, at least consciously, because they lack the emotional empathy and sense of responsibility for their behavior that triggers guilt. But, as we have discussed, they are tormented by shame.

Being fundamentally ashamed of themselves, people with NPD are experts at playing the shame game with those around them. Shaming others is narcissists' way of exorcising their pain. By planting shame in other people, narcissists in essence install a button they can press at any time to manipulate and punish those they seek to control. Those who love, care about, or otherwise look up to or rely on narcissists, such as their children, partners, relatives, friends, employees, students, congregants, or others within their sphere of influence, are vulnerable to messages of shame. Because narcissists do not feel remorse for hurting people and abusing their power over others, but in fact believe they are justified in doing so, they shame with abandon.

Children of narcissists are most vulnerable to being shamed because they are unformed beings who naturally love their parents and look to them for caregiving, validation of self, and a sense of identity. A shamed child often carries false and deeply damaging self-beliefs for decades, if not a lifetime.

Narcissists shame others in seemingly endless ways, from the commonplace to the bizarre, and very often with no basis in reality. For example, a very intelligent child may be shamed as stupid. In fact, narcissists often shame others for things that are actually their strengths, as a way to weaken them. And they often shame others as projections of things they themselves feel ashamed about, consciously or unconsciously, or about vulnerabilities they perceive in others. Possible sources of shame are myriad, but here are some common things narcissists shame others about being: angry, selfish, ugly, stupid, fat, emotional, clumsy, naive, lazy, self-indulgent, picky, promiscuous, unhelpful, unpopular, nonathletic, disloyal, weak, incompetent, mean, careless, uncooperative, unreasonable, stubborn, sensitive, ungrateful, and the list goes on.

Consequences of Shame

Shame is a powerfully destabilizing emotion that can be emotionally crippling. For anyone, intense shame can lead to:

1. Pervasive anxiety and panic attacks
2. Self-hatred
3. Withdrawal and secrecy
4. Fear of intimacy and "exposure"

5. Addictions
6. Self-harm
7. Internalized or externalized anger
8. Dislocation from one's feelings or authentic self
9. Perfectionism
10. Self-sabotage and underachievement

Narcissists ingrain shame in such a way that *you* end up doing the work of distrusting and hating yourself *for them.*

WEIGHT-LOSS CAMPAIGN

When Peggy was 14, her father, a professor, told her she needed to lose weight. To help "motivate" her, he convinced one of his graduate students, an obese man in his late twenties, to go on a competing diet with her. During weekly weigh-ins, Peggy and the graduate student would get on a scale and Peggy's father would mock whomever had lost less weight and give $5 to the "winner," pointing out how generous he was. <<

GASLIGHTING

The term *gaslighting* comes from the 1944 Hollywood film *Gaslight*, in which a husband dims the gaslights to make his wife believe she is going insane. Gaslighting is an insidious form of psychological manipulation meant to undermine a person's confidence in his or her perceptions of reality. The gaslighter uses suggestion, insinuation, dismissal, denial, and false claims to erode another person's belief in his or her own ability to interpret, judge, remember, and/or otherwise make sense of situations. Whereas a smear campaign is intended to erode someone's credibility with others, gaslighting is meant to erode someone's credibility with him- or herself. The narcissistic personality gaslights others fundamentally to weaken their position and strengthen her/his own. Because narcissists may be careful to gaslight within the scope of plausible deniability and away from witnesses, recognizing their abuse and calling it out can be difficult. Gaslighting enables the narcissist to:

1. Appear right
2. Appear reasonable
3. Feel superior
4. Play the victim
5. Assert control
6. Win arguments
7. Shift blame
8. Get her/his way
9. Avoid accountability
10. Get away with abuse

Gaslighting may be as simple as denying things that were said or claiming things happened when they didn't. After an abusive incident, a gaslighting narcissist may dismiss the abuse as unintended or harmless, outright deny that the abuse took place, or blame the abused. A cheating spouse, for example, may dismiss and deny evidence of an affair while accusing his or her partner of doing the cheating. Gaslighters often use *you* statements. They say things like the following:

- "It's always something with you."
- "You're being paranoid."
- "You're too sensitive."
- "Why do you doubt me all the time?"
- "You don't believe in me."
- "You're exaggerating again."
- "You can't possibly believe that."
- "You're always confused."
- "Can't you let go of the past?"
- "You're being irrational."
- "You need a shrink."
- "You have no sense of humor."
- "I can't help it if you can't remember anything."
- "What does it take to win with you?"
- "You're crazy."
- "You never listen."
- "Can you hear yourself?"

- "Can't you take a joke?"
- "You started it."
- "You never let anything go."
- "Whatever you say."
- "You're naive."
- "You need to get over it already."
- "You made me do that."
- "It's not my fault that you don't remember anything."

Parents in narcissistic families often gaslight their children about their personality, feelings, past behavior, and/or relationships as a way to disarm them, distort their self-image, and create self-doubt. Scapegoated children are typically sent the message in direct and indirect ways that their point of view is without merit, their feelings are unfounded, and they are to blame for family problems. Such parents may say things like the following:

- "I try to teach you, but you never learn."
- "You don't really feel that."
- "You've always been angry."
- "There is no pleasing you."
- "You have unreasonable expectations."
- "You never did learn to let things go."
- "You're an impossible child."
- "You're the reason your father/mother is never around."
- "Good girls/boys don't act like you do."
- "I don't know how you got this way."
- "Your sister/brother would never say that."
- "I do everything for you, and it's never enough."

Gaslighting may happen sporadically or occur routinely in a systematic process. In the most extreme cases, a gaslighter may be conducting a calculated, ongoing campaign to make another person believe s/he is losing her/his hold on reality.

The best defense against gaslighting is a secure belief in your own perceptions, something that can be difficult to achieve if you have been raised with undermining messages. However, once you understand what gaslighting is, how it works, and how to recognize it in your relationships, you can begin to separate yourself from the patterns. Although the narcissist will rarely if ever admit to gaslighting, once you stop reacting to it and show that it has no power over you, it is likely to end.

TRIANGULATING

Triangulation is another common form of manipulation in the narcissistic family. When someone triangulates, s/he interferes in relationships or brings a third party into a situation to gain leverage. Through triangulation, the narcissist controls the content and exchange of communication, takes things out of context, spreads distortions and lies, sets up implied or direct negative comparisons, and instigates rivalries between others. A closet narcissist father, for example, triangulates his wife and son by telling her that their son complains to him about what a controlling mother she is, while telling their son that she complains to him about what a difficult son he is. He uses triangulation to stir up insecurity and conflict between them that weakens their relationship and makes him appear like the better parent. Perhaps there is an existing point of contention between mother and son that makes his claims seem credible. Once rifts are established, he only needs to use occasional triangulation to produce ongoing discord between them and gain the upper hand.

Triangulation is a normal part of human dynamics that isn't necessarily meant to harm. To understand triangulation, it is important to look at it in context, consider the source, and examine the intent behind it. For example, a loving parent's comment about a difference between siblings may be innocent, whereas a narcissistic parent's comment may be intended to incite insecurity and jealousy.

Triangulation is often the norm in the narcissistic home, where direct communication is continuously undermined. By triangulating, narcissistic parents and/or narcissistic siblings wield control over family relationships, orchestrating drama and fanning flames of doubt and distrust. The best way to respond to triangulation is to dismantle it by communicating directly with the other person in the triangle or declining to discuss others with the narcissist and her/his flying monkeys. This can be difficult in families where bonds are already strained and insecurities rule interactions. But because narcissists rely on creating division and alienation between others, removing their influence can be an effective way to shift the power dynamic and repair broken connections in the family.

CONTRAST AND COMPARE

In Peter's family, his mother frequently triangulated him and his brother Jon. "It seemed like everything was either a direct or implied comparison between us," Peter said. His mother often set up competitions between the kids, such as who could name a state capital or remember a historic fact. Whoever came up with the right answer first got praised. "Usually Jon was the winner, because he was older. Even when Jon wasn't around, Mom always seemed to be comparing us. She'd say, 'No one is as special as Jon' or 'Jon is a person of rare gifts,' and I always knew the other side of the coin was that I wasn't those things," Peter said. <<

COGNITIVE DISTORTIONS

People with NPD by definition have cognitive distortions that interfere with their ability to reason, see middle ground, judge fairly, act impartially, and moderate their emotions. As parents, they model irrational thinking patterns and often dogmatically insist that their children agree with them. Cognitive distortions go hand in hand with emotional reactivity and lead to misunderstanding and misinformation.

Here are several forms of cognitive distortion common in narcissistic families:

1. False Dichotomies

The narcissist's either/or thinking creates false dichotomies, or the belief that only two sides of an issue are possible and that one must be right and the other wrong. Narcissistic parents have this reductionist view and expect their kids to go along with it. They typically categorize their children and view things as mutually exclusive. If one child is good at math, for example, the other must be bad at it. Or if the family identifies as high-achieving, then everyone must fall in line with talent and success. Children in these situations are forced into roles. They often struggle with the confused belief that to be loyal to one parent they must reject the other, which naturally causes anguish, confusion, alienation, and guilt. They may also feel forced to take sides between their siblings and other relatives, their friends, and even parts of themselves such as feminine or masculine, creative or logical, and athletic or studious.

Example: "Martha is the brains of the family! She gets straight A's. Jesse hasn't started school yet, but we can tell he'll be the athlete."

2. Personalizing

It is natural to personalize our experience somewhat through our own point of view. But narcissists habitually relate external events and situations back to themselves and often assume that others' thoughts or actions are somehow personally targeted at them. This exacerbates their emotional reactivity and breeds misunderstanding and paranoia.

Example: "The Morrisons keep those old cars in the yard just to spite me!"

3. Filtering

When we engage in filtered thinking, we focus on certain details we're looking for and downplay or ignore ones that don't match our bias. Narcissists are prone to filtering to support their view of themselves and others and to justify their behavior. Filtering is often "negative" or "positive" depending on narcissists' emotional state.

Example: "Jake has everything, and I have nothing. His boys are handsome, his house is perfect, and after his wife died, everyone felt sorry for him."

4. Polarized Thinking

Polarized thinking involves seeing things in extremes with little to no middle ground. Narcissists never learned to integrate positive and negative aspects of themselves or others into a realistic perception.

Example: "No other city compares with New York, and no other people compare with New Yorkers. The biggest and brightest come here because anything and everything that matters happens in New York."

5. Overgeneralizing

When we overgeneralize, or stereotype, we take one or a few isolated examples and generalize them into a fact or larger pattern without adequate evidence. Narcissists tend to overgeneralize for the same reason they use polarized thinking—because they miss complexity and interpret reality to match their overriding emotional needs.

Example: "She didn't hire me because she's a lesbian, and everyone knows that lesbians hate men."

6. Catastrophizing

When we catastrophize, we worry about things that might happen, look for trouble, interpret things negatively, assume the worst, and jump to worst-case scenarios. Life becomes a minefield where small or insignificant things are inflated into potential disasters, insurmountable obstacles, or exaggerated losses. Narcissists may catastrophize because they want attention and sympathy, need to see themselves as victims, or are easily overwhelmed by anxiety.

Example: "I've been up all night worrying that it might snow this weekend, which will mean my flight will be canceled and I'll be stuck at the airport and miss Thanksgiving."

7. Minimizing

The flip side of catastrophizing, minimizing involves denying or dismissing real issues or problems. Narcissists routinely minimize their abusive behavior to deflect responsibility and blame. And they minimize other people's concerns or problems, such as a child's hurt feelings, so they don't have to deal with them.

Example: "The kid is too sensitive. I needed to get his attention, so I raised my voice and I guess it startled him, but I don't see why he would cry about it."

SMEAR CAMPAIGNS

A smear campaign is an organized, intentional form of character assassination designed to discredit someone within his or her family, social circle, community, profession, or even the public at large. Smear campaigns happen in many settings, such as politics or places of business. They are often irresistible to narcissists as a way to:

1. Justify their actions
2. Control the narrative
3. Mount a preemptive strike
4. Influence others to take their side
5. Play the victim
6. Get the upper hand
7. Derive sadistic enjoyment
8. Sabotage a "competitor"
9. Punish
10. Look superior

Narcissists may smear another person because that person knows things they don't want known, they are trying to shift blame for their own bad behavior, or they are taking revenge. They also may conduct a smear campaign for lesser reasons, such as jealousy, resentment, or small slights. Whatever the reason, narcissists, lacking a moral compass, can be quite calculating and ruthless in discrediting and socially isolating a target. They may use innuendo, gossip, distortions, omissions, and outright lies to cast doubt and blame where it does not belong. A narcissist may smear an ex to their children, a scapegoated child to relatives and friends, or a colleague to other colleagues. The smear campaign usually happens behind the target's back and often with the assistance of the narcissist's enablers/flying monkeys.

TWILIGHT ZONE

Zora had been with Cher for ten years and shared a house and dog with her. When Zora started gaming with people online, Cher acted jealous and worried that she was cheating, despite Zora's reassurances that she wasn't. After months of fighting about Zora's nonexistent infidelity, Zora came home one evening from work to find that her key wouldn't open the front door. "I thought there was something wrong with the lock," she recalled. "I knew Cher was inside, so

I pounded on the door. She texted me that she had changed the locks and refused to speak to me. I started calling friends and learned that she had told our social circle that I was cheating on her. She had even gone to my family, and they were questioning my side of the story." Devastated and ashamed, Zora isolated herself, only talking with friends at work and her therapist. "It was like a *Twilight Zone* episode, where your life as you know it falls out from under your feet," Zora said. "In the end, Cher was the one who left me for someone else, but most people still believed I had caused the breakup. I realized she had been cheating on me all along, and the whole thing was an elaborate smear campaign so she wouldn't look like the bad guy for leaving me." <<

SUICIDE AND OTHER TRAGEDIES

Sometimes the trauma of life in a narcissistic home leads to tragedy, such as institutionalization, overdose, criminality, homelessness, and suicide. Parents may pathologize a scapegoated child to the point of institutionalizing or disowning that child. Some children are driven to levels of despair, rage, and dysfunction that result in mental illness, disability, serious or fatal accidents, prison, or suicide. Exes in combative divorce scenarios may be stripped of financial resources, suffer social ostracism, lose child custody, or face parental alienation. For family members, such realities are nothing short of devastating, adding to the trauma and making the need to find support for healing that much more important.

TWO GENERATIONS OF SCAPEGOATS

Matt was well aware that his father was an abusive narcissist, but he wanted to understand why his mother had married him and gone along with it. When he looked into her past, he learned that her father was narcissistic, too, and she had been his golden child. Matt also discovered that his mother had had a brother who was institutionalized most of his life. "They never gave him a firm diagnosis. Some said he had a borderline personality, some said he had severe PTSD. I think the truth was that he had been the family scapegoat, and my grandparents put him in a mental facility for it," Matt said. "The chilling thing is that my parents did the same thing to my brother. He was the sweetest kid, but Dad was always riding him, and they institutionalized him for a while when he was a teenager. Our mother got him out, but he's never been a functional adult." <<

THE NARCISSIST'S VIOLENT RAGE: A DAMAGE LIST FROM SURVIVORS

"A car windshield and the grocery cart he threw into it" —SUE

"He drove a $25,000 John Deere tractor through the garage door." —AVA

"My wall-to-wall living room window" —DARIUS

"He smashed my MacBook Pro on the floor in front of our children when I didn't take his food out of the oven in time." —ADRIENNE

"He killed my cat." —SURYA

"A ceiling fan with the barstool that he also broke" —TASTEE

"Empty wine bottles" —ROSEMARY

"He smashed an acoustic guitar on our street and left it there." —FAITH

"After I confronted him about suspected infidelity, he broke the dining room table by throwing it across the room and then hurled a coffee cup right through the oven door. And yes, he was cheating, again." —TAMMY

"She broke my will to live." —SAMUEL

"My ex once punched a hole in the wall and then ripped the entire 4 x 8-foot sheet of drywall down. I'm excellent at drywall work, thanks to him." —MARY

"I lost count of how many cell phones." —DANI

"My heart, my soul, my self-esteem, my happiness, my confidence" —TANIA

"His favorite 'throw' was throwing my daughter and me out of the house in the cold." —REBECCA

"He burnt all my clothes, punched holes in doors, emptied bank accounts." —MEG

"She ripped up my journals." —BARB

"A pole over my head" —GLEN

"My dog's ribs" —BETTY

"He threw out my dad's ashes." —JEN

"He broke his hand from punching the wall." —MINDY

"Our children's toys" —SONDRA

"My ribs, feet, jaw, fingers, kneecaps, eye socket, teeth, and nose . . . but never my will to survive" —KATT

ten

Chasing the Narcissist's Respect and Love

T HOSE OF US CLOSE TO PEOPLE WITH A NARCISSISTIC PERSONALITY DIS-
order (NPD) naturally find ourselves wondering, even obsessing over, what they care about and respect, which often seems arbitrary, contradictory, and fleeting. Family, friends, and anyone else within the narcissist's orbit are driven to search, both consciously and unconsciously, for answers about how to earn that person's elusive respect and love in an effort to connect, receive approval, and avoid conflict.

THE NARCISSIST'S "RESPECT"

We tell ourselves that, deep down, narcissists must care about dignity, kindness, truth, mercy, justice, compassion, gratitude, and love. Why wouldn't they? These are fundamental codes that define our best selves, ideals we aspire to and build relationships, families, institutions, and societies upon. We may fall short, but most of us recognize the importance and rewards of reaching toward these goals. Narcissists themselves often say they believe in such ideals, holding themselves up as paragons of principle and virtue.

We think that if we act with compassion, honesty, and integrity, the narcissists in our lives will recognize our honorable intentions and respect them. We think that if we are fair, they will be fair. If we are compassionate toward them, they will be compassionate toward us. If we care about their well-being, they will care about ours. If we love them, they will love us.

Sadly, the reality is that narcissistically disordered people do not reciprocate goodwill and rarely sustain respect for anything. Their hierarchical all-or-nothing thinking adds up to a harshly cynical world view of winners and losers. Their excessive sense of entitlement justifies violating the rights of those they view as less entitled. Their need to feel superior leads them to mistreat others as inferiors. And their lack of emotional empathy often amounts to cruel and destructive treatment of anyone in their path.

So, how about respecting power, wealth, fame, and influence? The answer? Although narcissists idealize people and things they believe will enhance their own status, they are driven by a desire to possess and control such coveted prizes. Typically, once winners are won over, they cease to live up to the narcissist's larger-than-life standards and are relegated to the worthless disappointment bin. Disillusion and devaluation follow narcissists' unrealistic expectations. If narcissists are thwarted in getting what they want, they are inclined to feel envy and a desire to debase and/or destroy what they cannot have. The unattainable becomes something to be outdone and defeated until no one but the narcissist stands tall.

THE NARCISSIST'S CONTEMPT

The bottom line is that narcissists nearly inevitably reach a point of contempt about everyone and everything. If that sounds extreme, consider a dictionary definition of *contempt*: "the feeling that a person or a thing is beneath consideration, worthless, or deserving scorn." Ultimately, virtually nothing and no one is spared the narcissist's cynical contempt.

People with NPD have contempt for:
1. **Language**, which they twist and distort
2. **Kindness**, which they see as disingenuous or gullible weakness
3. **Honesty**, which they avoid and subvert
4. **Responsibility**, which they deflect onto others
5. **Trust**, which they violate
6. **Love**, which they do not consistently feel but use as a weapon against others who do

7. **Authenticity**, which threatens their facade
8. **Generosity**, which threatens their primitive selfishness
9. **Forgiveness**, which they regard as admitting fault and giving others power
10. **Remorse**, which they do not feel but see as weakness in others to be exploited
11. **Accuracy**, which threatens their self-protective distortions of reality
12. **Truth**, which they fear and work to deny, dismiss, and deform

THE NARCISSIST'S "LOVE"

Whether you see the relationship with the narcissist in your life as a loving one is a matter of how extreme that person's personality impairment is, what your needs are in the relationship, and how you define love. We all have strengths and weaknesses and somewhat different ways of expressing and experiencing love. And love itself takes many forms. It can be steady or mercurial, short-term or long-lasting, romantic or platonic. Even so-called unconditional love usually in reality carries some conditions. Someone we have loved deeply may cross lines that are unacceptable to us, such as becoming physically violent, lying about something important, or succumbing to destructive addiction. But for most of us, the kind of love we hope to give and receive—love that is intimate and based on mutual acceptance, affection, respect, and continued growth—is probably not the kind of love we will ever share with a narcissistic personality. Certainly the child's fundamental need for unconditional loving validation is well beyond a narcissist's capabilities.

Narcissists place their needs first and habitually devalue and harshly reject those most close to them, something emotionally healthy and empathetic people do not do, even if they wish to end a relationship. For partners/spouses, such treatment often occurs after a period of idealization that may feel euphoric. Such people often stay in miserable relationships with narcissists far beyond all reason and self-respect, struggling to regain the initial "love-bombing" they experienced early in the relationship. Often, they blame themselves for the narcissist's devaluation and may even crave a return to the relationship that has ended brutally.

To children and adult children, a narcissistic parent frequently doles out positive attention as intermittent reinforcement interspersed with neglect and abuse, keeping them guessing and working for validation. This treatment on the part of the narcissist can be intentional or unconscious. Such children may seek approval for decades, even a lifetime, enduring excruciating indifference and/or punishment, perhaps with occasional moments or periods of acknowledgment, affection, concern, and generosity. It is common for adult children of narcissists to carry a fantasy that someday their parents will finally admit their abuses and open their arms with the love such children have sought their entire lives, to no avail. Although this fantasy is particularly resonant for scapegoated and ignored children, even so-called golden children, hero children, and mascots understand that their narcissistic parent's "love" is conditional, something they must continually work to uphold or lose. Both scapegoated and favored children are not recognized or valued for their authentic selves but instead for how they can serve the narcissistic parent's needs, whether as negative or positive projections.

There may be proclamations of love and concern, even intermittent caring gestures, but by definition, narcissists are pathologically self-serving and abusively devaluing of others. Their extremist, hierarchical thinking and unstable self-esteem make them rigid and harshly demanding. And their impaired empathy means that they do not consistently, if ever, emotionally engage with others beyond seeking something they want.

BAIT AND SWITCH

Adelle described her father as a seasoned psychologist with a serial history of seducing and then dumping women, some of whom were his clients and all of whom were younger and more attractive than him. "My father is not and never has been a good-looking man," Adelle said, "but he has an absolute tried-and-true process with women. He listens very carefully to what they really want and need in their lives and then supports it 1,000 percent—at first." Adelle recalled that starting when she was about 13, after her parents divorced, her father would introduce her to each new woman in his life the same way. "He'd tell me in front of her, very charmingly, that I *had to love her* and that she was *true family*, something he always implied I was not." Adelle explained that after each new conquest fell in love with him, he would raise the price tag for his attention. "He required them to provide more adulation and tolerate more derision. The wonderful promise would be increasingly withheld as they became desperate," explained Adelle. "I always knew when he was about to break up a relationship. He'd say the exact same thing: 'I wish I had known how emotionally unbalanced she was.'" ‹‹

THE RULES DON'T APPLY TO ME

Lucia's mother-in-law, Elaine, prided herself on getting around rules. After her husband died, she continued to display his "handicapped" placard in her car so she could park near building entrances. She would even fake a limp to appear disabled. After Lucia was paralyzed in an accident, she began relying on handicapped spots. One day as she was looking for a parking place at the grocery store, she recognized Elaine's car parked in a disabled spot. "I knew Elaine had been doing this, and here it was in my face," she said. "When I saw her in the store, I tried to explain to her that what she was doing affected other people. She didn't apologize and kept using the sign until it expired. That really helped me understand what my husband went through growing up." ‹‹

eleven

Why Narcissism Runs in Families

I F YOU'RE SEEING A RECURRING PATTERN OF NARCISSISTIC PEOPLE APPEAR-
ing in your life, there are reasons narcissism may be clustering around you
and cause for hope that you can end the cycle.

You may have heard of disease clusters, where certain diseases or disorders occur in an unusually high incidence in close proximity. NPD is no
exception to this phenomenon, with clusters happening in families across
generations and connected through both biology and marriage.

NARCISSISM IS YOUR NORMAL

If you've grown up with one or more narcissistic parents or stepparents,
sadly, narcissism may be your normal. The familiar is a powerful force for
most of us (even and especially unconsciously), and you may find yourself
drawn by and to further narcissists, as friends, bosses, employees, romantic partners, and even doctors and therapists. The narcissist's projection,
gaslighting, and belittlement are all too familiar to you, and you've been
groomed to take abuse and blame yourself for it in the process. If you were
scapegoated by a domineering narcissistic father, for example, chances are
you will wear a kick-me sign on your back in future relationships until you
learn to find a healthier new normal.

The Good News: Regardless of what you grew up with, narcissism is not
normal. Unlike narcissists, most people develop relatively stable selfhood,
learn emotional empathy, and possess a reasonable moral compass that guides

them in their relationships. Growing up under the shadow of NPD by no means dooms you to develop the disorder, nor does it mean you must repeat its patterns. However, it does predispose you to further narcissistic relationships until you actively work to change your life. Examining your family of origin, educating yourself about the diseased roots and destructive patterns of narcissism, and becoming self-aware in your relationships are powerful steps to break its grip over your life. Learn more about codependency in Chapter 13.

MONKEY SEE, MONKEY DO

Like all primates, humans learn from others, particularly caregivers such as parents, grandparents, and older siblings. If you have narcissistic models, you are likely to repeat at least some narcissistic patterns of thinking, feeling, and behaving. You may pick up your narcissistic parent's traits and become narcissistic yourself, perpetrating on others the negation of self you endured. You may emulate an enabling parent and find yourself acting as a codependent to a narcissistic partner. Or you may raise a narcissistic child, unwittingly creating an unhealthy environment like the one you grew up in and possibly passing along a genetic predisposition to NPD.

The Good News: Primates, particularly humans, are highly adaptive animals with flexibility and the capacity to continue learning throughout life. Poor modeling in your family of origin can be overcome and replaced with healthy patterns. Just because your family of origin had narcissists does not mean you are destined to be narcissistic as well. The influence of good models, for example in the form of an emotionally stable other parent, relative, friend, and/or teacher, can be a powerfully transformative force for good. And bad examples often provide the most lasting lessons.

BIOLOGY

As we have discussed, disruptions in attachment with primary caregivers have long been seen as the likely cause of NPD. However, genetic and neurobiological influences are also increasingly recognized in the development of the disorder. As with many conditions, such as alcoholism or schizophrenia, a combination of nurture and nature is most likely at work in a child developing narcissistic adaptations that progress into full-blown NPD in adulthood.

The Good News: A healthy, resilient connection between children and their caregivers may turn off the genetic switches in a young person's DNA that influence the development of NPD.

GENERATIONAL TRAUMA

Tragically, narcissism is often the radioactive gift that keeps on giving from one generation to the next. A narcissistic mother may pass on her NPD to her son, who repeats the pattern through distorted behaviors with his own children, who in turn continue the cycle with their children. Like attracts like, and trauma in one form or another has a way of repeating itself. Even a child from a narcissistic family who does not develop narcissism may marry a partner with the disorder and continue patterns with his or her own children, increasing the likelihood of perpetuating the damage in future generations.

The Good News: Although by definition generational trauma tends to ripple forward, it is by no means a foregone conclusion. New generations bring different parents, parenting styles, social influences, and genetics into play that all offer opportunities for healthier outcomes. Most living beings by nature move toward light and healing, choosing peace over discord and love over cruelty and hate. Once you know and recognize what you're dealing with, you have the power to heal.

PART 4

PARTNERS OF NARCISSISTS

Romance, Partnership, and Breakup with a Narcissist

I**T IS EASY TO GET IN THICK WITH A NARCISSIST. PRONE TO INFATUATION** and dependent on others for their emotional survival, people with NPD are driven to find the "perfect" mate and can be exceptionally persistent in pursuing a love interest.

ROMANTIC IDEALIZATION

Given to extremes and lacking healthy boundaries, narcissists tend to go all in during the early stages of romance. When they meet someone who seems ideal, they elevate and typically "love bomb" that person with extravagant interest in the form of excessive attentiveness and flattery, abrupt expressions of intimacy, and premature declarations of love and commitment. One of the narcissist's main forms of seduction is mirroring.

Mirroring

Mirroring, or reflecting back what others say and do, is a common behavior that many of us engage in, often unconsciously, to create rapport and show feelings of connectedness with others. We may, for example, adopt another person's (or animal's) energy level, tone, facial expressions, and body language to show understanding, reassurance, and empathy.

People with NPD, conversely, use mirroring in place of empathy. With a prospective or new partner, they reflect back that person's style, interests, and values. If you like gardening, artisanal chocolate, and crossword puzzles, so do they! If you're into tattoos, suddenly they show up with one. If you want five kids, wow, they do, too.

Narcissists mirror for three primary reasons:

1. They lack a stable identity and are trying on yours.
2. They are working to win you over, reflecting back what they think you want to see.
3. They are mimicking intimacy, because they lack the capacity for genuine deep connection.

If you are on the receiving end of this kind of attention, it can feel like you've met your soulmate—someone who has the same likes and dislikes, the same take on life. If you have been romanced by a narcissist, you know that initially they work to hone in on your deepest needs and vulnerabilities[1] and devote themselves to fulfilling your desires. In this idealization phase, the narcissist's infatuated intensity may make you feel as if you have found "the one." Because this can be intoxicating, the narcissist's attentions may lead you to ignore your better judgment and usual caution.

DEVALUATION AND DISCARD

But being prone to simplistic all-or-nothing thinking and an insistence on unattainable perfection, narcissists in relationships inevitably become disenchanted and rejecting. And because they lack a moral compass, they do not hesitate to express their disappointment in a range of hostile behaviors, including complaints, demands, denigration, mind games, and rationalizations for rage, if not outright betrayal and abandonment.

Narcissists in romantic relationships nearly always reach the devaluation phase, but they do not necessarily discard. Some jump from one conquest to the next, but many seek out and remain in long-term relationships, typically treating their partner to an ongoing host of manipulations and abuses. The narcissistic spouse also may alternate idealizing and devaluing treatment as a means of control or because s/he is vacillating emotionally.

People in long-term relationships with narcissistic partners are expected to do the following endlessly and with little to no reciprocation:

1. Mind read
2. Agree without question
3. Acquiesce without hesitation
4. Self-sacrifice
5. Give attention
6. Give admiration
7. Clean up literal and figurative messes that are not their own
8. Excuse callous and abusive behavior
9. Endure constant criticism
10. Submit to boundary violations
11. Accept double standards
12. Provide reassurance
13. Forgive transgressions
14. Defer their needs
15. Take the blame for how the narcissist has hurt them

It's not personal; it's the narcissist's way.

WHY YOU DIDN'T SEE IT COMING

Because individuals with NPD see life in childlike terms, they view love interests unrealistically, either as perfect mates or worthless disappointments. But in the early stages of romance, their idealizing attentions can make it difficult for others to see their binary thinking and lack of empathy until after they have done profound harm.

Anyone can get tripped up in a relationship with a narcissist. Narcissism is so insidiously toxic and far beyond the normal bounds of human conscience and decency that it is virtually impossible to imagine or understand unless you have lived with it firsthand. The fact that narcissists often calculatingly hide their haughty and degrading attitude when it suits them and use all manner of manipulation to project their abuses onto those they abuse makes it all the harder to see through the madness.

LIFE WITH THE NARCISSIST: HELL IN A HAMSTER WHEEL

If you are still with your narcissistic partner after the idealization phase, your entangled relationship is probably littered with broken promises, cruelties, regrets, and possibly financial and legal woes. Having been treated to painful devaluation, you feel like an emotionally shattered soldier fighting to survive and, if you have kids, to help them survive. Your relationship is hell in a hamster wheel, with you running to stay sane and escape the daily abuse but never actually getting anywhere, only more trapped and exhausted. You are caught in the narcissist's alternative reality, a violent distortion of the truth that serves her/his need to feel exceptional and entitled at everyone else's expense.

Narcissists need you far more than you need them, but they will never let you know that. They are so fearful of having their narcissistic injury triggered and so preemptively attacking and vicious that they will continue to abuse you as long as you allow them to. Although you may long for escape, you may also miss your narcissistic partner's original seductive attention and adulation. You may love his or her good qualities and wonder what you can do to regain his or her love.

But as much as you may care about your partner and your relationship, the narcissist in your life only sees you through a myopic lens of "what's in it for me?" Narcissists cannot truly care about anyone's needs but their own. They are essentially a destructive parasite, and as long as you stay in a relationship with a narcissist, you are her/his enabling host, sacrificing your happiness, stability, self-esteem, and emotional and physical well-being for someone incapable of reciprocating your love.

Elinor Greenberg describes the narcissistic partner this way:

Narcissists rarely feel any genuine warmth for anybody but themselves and the current object of their admiration. What passes for warmth by a Narcissist is either a calculated act intended to deceive others and get the Narcissist what he or she wants; or a basking in the pleasurable way someone else's admiration is currently making the Narcissist feel. Thus, when a Narcissist says: "I love you," what he or she *really* means is: "I love the way you are making me feel about me right now." Moreover, since people are usually totally interchangeable to most Narcissists, the current recipient of their positive feelings can quickly be deposed if circumstances dictate.[2]

PERSONALITY TYPES WHO FALL FOR NARCISSISTS

Anyone can end up in a romantic relationship with a narcissist. But there are personality types more likely than most to attract and be attracted to narcissists as well as more likely to stay in such relationships against their best interests.

1. You Were Raised by Narcissists

As someone raised by one or more narcissistic parents/stepparents, your normal is a narcissistic relational dynamic. Whether you were a golden child or scapegoat, lost child or mascot, you are susceptible to falling into romantic relationships or marriages with narcissists. In your family, your parents modeled this for you and you were thrust into a codependent role that you are likely to repeat until you recognize the pattern and actively work to change it. It is common to replay familiar life roles. We are often emotionally and physiologically programmed to do so. But the good news is that you can break your pattern with narcissists, learn to overcome, and move on.

2. You Were Raised in Other Traumatic Circumstances

Children raised in other types of dysfunctional environments, such as a family dominated by addiction or an abusive foster care situation, may be predisposed to accept and even seek out narcissistic relationships. People with low self-esteem as a result of traumatic childhood experiences, including psycho-emotional, physical, and/or sexual violation, are vulnerable to narcissists. Early trauma may have left you with tendencies toward self-destruction and reenacting victimization. You may have received the message that you don't deserve decency, affection, boundaries, stability, or unconditional love. You may have few experiences with kindness, let alone love. Narcissists prey on vulnerable people who will bend to their will.

3. You Are Highly Empathic

As a person keenly attuned to others' emotions, you can be vulnerable to exploitation by people who lack empathy—a state of being that for most of us, and especially the very empathetic, is difficult to comprehend. Because of your sensitivity, you may be drawn to helping others who are emotionally needy and impaired, particularly the profoundly wounded narcissist.

4. You Are a Caretaker/Rescuer

You want to help, cure, restore, repair, protect, defend, and fight for what's right. You want to save people, animals, groups, and causes from harm and injustice. No matter the situation, you want to make things better. Chances are you grew up in a caretaking role of some kind and identify strongly as such, which can be both a gift and a trap depending on how well you have learned to establish healthy boundaries and balance your own needs with those of others.

You may view the narcissist in your life as your biggest challenge yet. But you alone cannot heal or cure people with NPD, and you cannot teach them empathy. They experienced disrupted attachment at a formative age and have profound developmental deficits. Maybe you can help them if they want to help themselves, and that's a big if. The question for you is, *Is it worth it?*

LOST BEST FRIEND

Nikki suffered from anxiety, but she never knew how much of it was coming from her or the stress of living with her boyfriend, who belittled her, fought with her mother, and dictated decisions. After Nikki gave birth to their daughter, she suffered a painful and lonely bout of postpartum depression. "My golden retriever Rex was always by my side. He would put his chin in my lap and comfort me while I cried, sometimes for hours," she said. "He was my best friend." After her boyfriend lost his job, although he still had income from his family and could afford payments on a new truck, he insisted that they give away Rex. "He told me we had to get rid of my dog because we couldn't afford vet bills if anything went wrong with his health," Nikki said. "He had always hated Rex. I never saw my dog again." <<

IS YOUR PARTNER A NARCISSIST?

Whether you are examining a current relationship or trying to make sense of a past one, it is understandably disturbing to think that you might have partnered with a narcissist. But facing that possibility is nowhere near as difficult as living with the reality of it. Asking the question, as painful as it is, is a necessary step toward empowering yourself.

If you have gotten this far as a reader, you probably already have your answer. But let's look at it head-on. Is your partner a narcissist? And, if so, how bad is it? Ask yourself the following questions.

How You Feel around Your Partner

1. Do you find yourself regularly placating your partner to avoid confrontation?
2. Do you hold back your opinions from your partner for fear of disagreement?
3. Are you frequently confused about what went wrong in your conversations with your partner?
4. Does it feel unsafe to freely express your feelings with your partner?
5. Do you hold back from sharing your thoughts for fear your partner will judge or disapprove?
6. Do you defer to your partner's wishes to avoid a fight?
7. Does it seem like you can never do anything right with your partner?
8. Are you regularly anxious or tense around your partner?
9. Do you feel you always say or do the wrong thing with your partner?
10. Do you edit what you tell your friends about your partner/relationship for fear it will look bad?
11. Do you find yourself making excuses for your partner's behavior?
12. Do you worry your partner will criticize or embarrass you in public?
13. Do you feel confident in other areas of your life but self-doubting around your partner?
14. Do you feel isolated by the relationship with your partner?
15. Do you limit contact with family or friends to avoid making your partner upset?
16. Do you frequently feel criticized and/or attacked by your partner?
17. Do you frequently feel guilty around your partner without knowing why?
18. Do you feel that everything comes down to what your partner wants?

19. Do you frequently wonder whether your partner loves you?
20. Do you feel physically unsafe around your partner?

How Your Partner Acts around You

21. Does your partner routinely interrupt or ignore you?
22. Does your partner constantly have to be center stage?
23. Is your partner hypersensitive but calls you too sensitive?
24. Is your partner frequently picky, irritable, and controlling about things you say and do?
25. Does your partner curse at you and call you names?
26. Does your partner berate you?
27. Does it feel as if your partner becomes a hostile stranger when you have a fight?
28. Does your partner act contemptuous of you?
29. Does your partner exaggerate or lie to you?
30. Does your partner say hurtful things that you would never say?
31. Does your partner use silent treatment to punish you?
32. Does your partner always seem to have the upper hand?
33. Does your partner blame you or others when things go wrong?
34. Does your partner act threatened or angry when you spend time with other people?
35. Is your partner combative with your family and/or friends?
36. Does your partner often interpret other people or situations differently than you do?
37. Does your partner threaten to leave you and take everything?
38. Is your partner physically violent?
39. Does your partner threaten or hurt you physically?
40. Does your partner hurt you again after promising to change?

If the answer to many or most of these questions is yes, you have good reason to think that your partner is narcissistic and abusive. If you are physically unsafe and/or feel regularly confronted with criticism, rage, and other forms of abuse, you owe it to yourself to try to find a way out. But be smart. If your partner is unstable and prone to blame and rage, you must take steps to protect yourself before confronting the situation or making other changes.

THE GOOD SOLDIER

As the emotional caretaker of his demanding and unstable mother, Cody took on codependent patterns and got into an abusive relationship in college. "For 12 years she lied to me, used me, and put me down behind my back, and I put up with it. After she got pregnant by another man, I helped her raise her daughter. I stayed because I believed she was the one. We planned to get married, but when I tried to address problems in our relationship she left. A month later, she married another guy. I was shattered." It wasn't until Cody learned about narcissism and codependency that he was able to process the past and let go emotionally. "I finally saw the big picture—how I was set up as a kid for self-sacrifice and neglecting my own needs," he said. "I'm still working on it, but now I understand what I don't want in a relationship." «

THE NARCISSIST AS HUMAN PARASITE

Looking at narcissism through the lens of parasitism helps us understand narcissists' reliance on others as a means of supply. Individuals with NPD are always seeking the attention and affirmation they did not receive at crucial developmental stages. Their incomplete sense of being compels them to seek self-worth externally. Narcissists as a human parasite take a heavy emotional and physiological toll on their "hosts."

Scientists have uncovered many parasite-host relationships in which the parasite actually alters the brain and behavior of its host to make it assist in fulfilling vital parts of the parasite's life cycle. A certain type of tiny wasp, for example, injects its egg along with chemicals into a ladybug.[3] The egg hatches and consumes the nutrients that the ladybug ingests when it eats, essentially devouring the ladybug from the inside out. When the wasp larva is big enough, it squirms out of the ladybug and wraps itself in a cocoon beneath it. Immobilized and half dead, the ladybug is still programmed in essence to protect the larva by thrashing its body around if threatening insects approach. Once the larva-turned-wasp hatches from its cocoon and flies away, the ladybug typically dies.

Like most parasites, narcissistically disordered people rarely kill their hosts, although malignant ones may subject them to violence or in extreme cases murder. But like the mind-altering variety of parasite, narcissists work to control the "brain" of their hosts through a wide range of manipulations, from bullying to gaslighting, projecting to victim-blaming, guilt-tripping to silent treatment. Narcissists continuously orchestrate the "reality" around themselves by enlisting others in supporting their delusions of grandeur and punishing and/or rejecting them if they do not comply. To narcissists, a spouse questioning an opinion they have declared as patented truth or their child not making the soccer team are potential humiliations to which they may react with scorn or rage. In parasitic narcissists' eyes, both situations weaken the desirability of their sources of supply and thereby threaten their sense of well-being.

Narcissists have an instinct for finding and attaching themselves to potential "hosts." Such people offer narcissists supply and often status while also enabling their harshly self-serving behavior and worldview. A host may confer status to the narcissist in many ways, such as by being well-liked, socially connected, educated, good looking, wealthy, famous, or professionally accomplished. The host also enables the narcissist by directly or indirectly being complicit in the narcissist's distorted reality and abusive behavior (such as by failing to confront that behavior or even by participating in it). In this sense, the enabling host is like the mind-altered ladybug, serving the needs of the narcissist, often at his or her own expense.

thirteen

Codependency and Narcissism

BEING FUNDAMENTALLY DEPENDENT ON OTHERS FOR THE SELF-ASSURANCE they lack, narcissists don't get very far without enablers. An enabling partner/spouse supports the narcissist's larger-than-life persona and accepts and perhaps even helps perpetrate his or her abusive behavior while also being victimized by it.

THE ENABLER/CODEPENDENT

People fall into enabling partnerships with narcissists for different reasons, from a desire to caretake, to self-doubt, to a need for approval. Often they become enablers gradually, without understanding their situation. They may feel confused by their partner's brainwashing messages, believing some or all of the following:

- I am causing her/him to act this way.
- I am the unfair/angry/cruel one.
- If I weren't so stupid/selfish/needy/unattractive, s/he would love me.
- S/he doesn't really mean to hurt me/the kids.
- Deep down s/he loves me/us but doesn't know how to show it.
- All relationships are difficult like this.
- Things will get better when we get married/have kids.
- If I change, s/he will be happy with me.
- If I am more loving/lovable, s/he will stop acting so angry.
- If our children act/do better, s/he will be happy with us.

Enablers may delude themselves into thinking that they alone can understand and fulfill their difficult but special partner. They may see their partner as somehow a great catch and believe they need to do extra work to keep him/her. Perhaps their partner feels a bit out of their league—more intelligent, attractive, charming, educated, or successful than they feel they are and therefore worth the high maintenance they need to do.

CODEPENDENT PATTERNS

As we discussed in Chapter 8, adult enablers typically accept abusive dynamics in a relationship with a narcissist because they grew up with demanding, selfish, neglectful, and/or abusive caregivers. In many cases, they themselves come from narcissistic homes, just as narcissists do. Or they experienced other dysfunctional family environments, such as ones dominated by religious extremism or addiction, in which they learned to subjugate their needs and feelings. Such people have developed codependent traits that draw them to narcissists and predispose them to reenacting early trauma and codependent patterns.

Just as narcissists are, codependents are characterized by common traits that reflect unhealthy and self-defeating ways of viewing themselves and relationships. Things that may have helped them cope in their families of origin hinder them in adulthood and lead to further trauma. Often coming from the same kind of family dysfunction, the narcissist and the codependent share several underlying problems. Like the narcissist, the codependent struggles with shame and alienation from his or her authentic self. Both have low self-esteem, poor boundaries, and a strong denial mechanism. Codependents also resemble narcissists in their tendency to tie their self-worth to others, take things personally, and feel victimized.

Traits Codependents Share with Narcissists

1. Dysfunctional family of origin
2. Low self-esteem
3. Underlying shame
4. Alienated from authentic self
5. Poor boundaries
6. Strong denial

7. Take things personally
8. Externalized self-worth
9. Imbalanced relationships
10. Feel victimized

But although codependents share traits with narcissists, codependents are also fundamentally different in ways that give them greater potential to overcome their self-destructive patterns and achieve personal well-being and healthier and more satisfying relationships. Before we look at ways to break out of codependency, let's look more closely at the codependent's mind-set.

Self-Defeating Codependent Traits

Children who grow into codependent adults learned to detach from their feelings and overvalue the feelings of others. They responded to their narcissistic parent's (or otherwise impaired parent's) inflated entitlement and constant demands by sublimating their needs and working overtime to please and appease that parent. In all likelihood, they learned this behavior from a codependent parent or other family member who modeled it. The codependent compensates for the narcissist's exaggerated *selfishness* with similarly exaggerated *selflessness*. In an unconscious effort to achieve balance in their family of origin and relationships, codependents sacrifice their own inner equilibrium.

Codependents tend to:

1. Dissociate from their feelings
2. Neglect their needs
3. Have an exaggerated sense of responsibility
4. Tie their self-worth and happiness to others
5. Fear being alone
6. Avoid their own problems by focusing on other people's problems
7. Derive self-esteem from helping/serving others
8. Give unsolicited advice and help
9. Give to the point of exhaustion
10. Believe they can control things beyond their control
11. Feel uncomfortable or guilty asking for help
12. Have difficulty knowing what they want
13. Accept blame for things not their fault

14. Feel they don't need or deserve caretaking
15. Mistake dependency and pity for love
16. Feel guilty for things that aren't their responsibility
17. Lie to themselves about their partner's behavior
18. Blame others for their partner's behavior
19. Believe they can rescue and/or fix their partner
20. Believe their partner can't cope without them

Although our society at times heroizes selflessness, it is not a healthy or sustainable way of being, and it is a dangerous thing to teach children. The codependent personality's compulsion to self-efface in service to others, particularly a domineering narcissist, is a setup for emptiness and victimization. Children raised by parents enacting such dynamics experience trauma and carry a blueprint for further dysfunction in their adult relationships. This is the definition of generational trauma, and its negative impact cannot be overstated. Parents who model self-alienation and denial, whether they be narcissistic or codependent, teach their kids to distrust their instincts, fear their emotions, and fight against their own best interests and the best interests of those around them. Shame rules the day, hurt begets more hurt, and potential for growth and connectedness is lost. As long as people enable narcissistic behavior and values, injustice follows and despair and suffering are the norm. You've heard it before, but it bears repeating: You can't help others without putting on your own oxygen mask first.

TRAUMA BONDING

Narcissists typically manipulate a codependent partner through alternating abuse and special treatment, which are often a reflection of the narcissists' fluctuating pattern of idealization and devaluation. The codependent falls into her/his own pattern of avoiding attack while also seeking such rewards as affection, praise, sex, or money. In this dynamic, the enabler experiences trauma bonding with the abusive narcissist, becoming emotionally and physically addicted to the roller coaster of positive and negative reinforcement.[1]

To outsiders, a trauma-bonded codependent partner may appear irrational and self-destructive for staying in the relationship. But the reality mirrors other forms of domestic abuse and can be very difficult to break free from because of the codependent's dysregulated trauma response. Often, such people are physiologically vulnerable to negative feedback loops of trauma-bonding addiction because of early experiences with narcissistic or otherwise inadequate caregiving in their family of origin. Bessel van der Kolk describes the process this way:

> When the persons who are supposed to be the sources of safety and nurturance become simultaneously the sources of danger against which protection is needed, children maneuver to re-establish some sense of safety. Instead of turning on their caregivers and thereby losing hope for protection, they blame themselves. They become fearfully and hungrily attached and anxiously obedient.[2]

As adults, such people are predisposed to unconsciously seek out and reenact patterns of abuse, with women more often playing the role of victim and men playing the role of aggressor.[3] Our cultural emphasis on male authority, privilege, and aggression and female subservience, service, and self-sacrifice both reflect and perpetuate toxic masculinity and destructive power imbalances at all levels of society. Whether one is in the role of selfish overtaker or selfless overgiver, alienation is the norm and self-actualization impossible. Regardless of gender or other markers of difference, we all need a balance of self-respect and humility, giving and receiving, intimacy and self-reliance, loving and letting go.

Frequently, codependent partners of narcissists stay in their relationships even when they realize they are being abused because they feel they deserve such treatment and/or don't see a way out. Their abusive mate is likely to have undermined their independence and support network by
  - eroding their self-confidence,
  - gaslighting their sense of reality,
  - burdening them with excessive responsibilities and problems,
  - isolating them from family and friends,
  - draining their finances,
  - alienating them from their children,
  - threatening to leave them with nothing, and/or
  - threatening to harm or even kill them.[4]

OVERCOMING CODEPENDENCY

But despite the deeply rooted trappings of codependency, there is a way out. Whereas narcissism is an entrenched condition extremely difficult to overcome, largely because the narcissist by definition believes s/he does not need to change,[5] codependency is much more amenable to treatment. Unlike the narcissist, the codependent usually has empathy, a strong sense of responsibility, a desire for intimacy, and willingness to help and support others. Building self-awareness and self-esteem are within reach for the codependent and are the keys to a healthier state of being and balanced relationships.

As a codependent, your vulnerabilities have the potential to become strengths. The path you took out of yourself to overfocus on others is the same path you can take back to yourself. You can use your

1. awareness of others' needs to become aware of your own,
2. empathy for others to feel compassion for yourself, and
3. desire to help and heal others to help and heal you.

Your first and biggest challenge as a codependent working to break free of defeating patterns is to give up your primitive denial defense. We have explored denial previously, and here we need some reminders. When parents are neglectful and/or abusive, young children must deny it to survive. They have no choice. But as they get older, eventually they must wake up from their denial so as to grow and heal. Children who don't break their denial get stuck, continue to get hurt, and end up hurting others. It's that simple, and that complicated.

One of the most difficult forms of denial to break is the belief that you can get the narcissist to love you. As we discuss throughout this book, narcissists do not reciprocate love, respect, compassion, concern, or caretaking. Narcissists want those things from you but cannot return them. *A narcissist does not feel what you feel, and you can't change that.*

But overcoming your denial is not enough. As a codependent, you must replace dysfunctional beliefs and patterns of behavior with more functional ones. This takes self-reflection, education, support, and lots and lots of practice. As you become honest with yourself, you reorient yourself with healthy alternatives to the ones you learned growing up. You move from codependence to interdependence in your relationships. You learn to:

1. Respect yourself
2. Listen to your needs
3. Value your feelings
4. Ask for what you want
5. Reject what you don't want
6. Separate your happiness from the happiness of others
7. Recognize imbalance in relationships
8. Establish healthy boundaries
9. Recognize your power and your limits
10. Let go of the need to control others
11. Let go of guilt and shame
12. Reparent yourself

We explore strategies for managing the narcissist in your life, processing your grief, asserting boundaries, and healing in Part 6.

 MARRYING YOUR FAMILY

Like so many who grow up in narcissistic families, Katy fell into a destructive relationship while still in her teens. After meeting her future husband as a pen pal, she was treated to love bombing and a marriage proposal before they had even met. "We fought constantly, but whenever we were apart, he would say we were soulmates and he couldn't live without me," Katy recalled. She agreed to marry him because she didn't think she deserved better. "It was years of physical abuse and screaming belittlement that would literally break me down to vomiting. I realize now that he just saw me as his meal ticket. He called me his paycheck with legs," she said.

In time, Katy grew stronger about setting boundaries. "Although he hated sex, he wanted to get me pregnant, but I refused. He assumed we'd have boys and would say it gave him a hard-on to think about having a son. What kind of person says that?" she said.

Nearly a decade after meeting, they finally divorced and Katy dated for a while, came out as bisexual, and found herself attracting narcissists of different genders. "By then, I was recognizing the signs and never allowed anything to get serious." She began to actively process her traumatic past and in time met her current partner, with whom she has had a loving relationship for the last 17 years. «

THE NARCISSIST AS NAKED EMPEROR

Many of the most enduring children's stories feature archetypal narcissistic characters, from the violent bullying of the Queen of Hearts in *Alice in Wonderland* and the callous abandoning mother bird in *Horton Hatches the Egg* to the grandiose blustering of the impostor wizard in *The Wizard of Oz.* Such stories reveal dark truths about adults and serve as cautionary tales against selfishness, deceit, and vanity. The fraudulent emperor in *The Emperor's New Clothes*,[6] a Hans Christian Andersen tale dating back nearly two hundred years to 1837, has powerful psychological lessons about narcissism and its societal grip.

The protagonist and literal naked butt of the story is the pompous emperor, who falls prey to con-artist self-proclaimed weavers of magic cloth. Promising they will sew the emperor a suit of clothes so fine it will be invisible to those who are "unfit for their positions, stupid, or incompetent," they exploit the emperor's narcissistic vanity, exaggerated entitlement, and desire for worshipful adoration. But most tellingly, they exploit his fear that he is a fraud: that he is in fact unfit, stupid, and incompetent. These are the narcissist's deepest self-beliefs, which he attempts to hide from himself and others at virtually any cost.

When the scammers present their "garment" to the emperor, it is nothing at all, literally thin air. They flatter and fawn over him as they pretend to fit him with his glorious new clothes, while he looks in the mirror and pretends to see what is not there. The emperor's advisers and servants play along out of self-doubt and fear of reprisal from their deluded ruler. When the emperor parades before the townspeople, they pretend as well. It is a child in the audience who finally declares the bald truth: "But he isn't wearing anything at all!"

The brilliance of the story, which has been translated into over one hundred languages, is the child's moment of revelation. Everyone sees the truth as plain as day, but the child's innocence and purity of vision compel him to declare it aloud for all to hear, breaking the spell of complicity among the adults.

As in the story, it is often children who question real-life narcissists. Confused by the dissonance between what they see and feel and what they are told is happening by their narcissistic and/or enabling parents, children naturally question the lies and denial that characterize life in a narcissistic home. Tragically, such children quickly learn that their honesty is considered sacrilege within their family and grounds for punishment. They are bullied and scapegoated into stuffing the truth and playing along with the narcissist's false alternate reality—one in which the narcissist is figuratively wearing magical clothes that make her/him superior, omnipotent, entitled, and deserving of adoration regardless of whether s/he does anything to deserve it.

Like the emperor's lackeys, enabling spouses and other family members are often manipulated and cowed into submission by the narcissist tyrant. Bullied, confused, and/or afraid of losing what power they have, they become complicit in upholding the narcissist's rule. Although they may agree with the child's uncorrupted awareness and sympathize with the child's position, they are too invested in the system to confront or leave the narcissist's reign. Unlike the child in the story, who is embraced by the town for speaking the truth, the truth-telling child in the narcissistic family is more often isolated, punished, or even banished from the kingdom.

fourteen

Staying with or Leaving Your Narcissistic Partner

W HETHER YOU CHOOSE TO STAY WITH OR LEAVE YOUR PARTNER IS YOUR decision and will depend on factors only you can evaluate. You will need to consider the consequences for yourself and for others involved such as children. Whatever choice you make, there are steps you can take to protect yourself and better manage your situation.

STAYING IN THE RELATIONSHIP

There are many reasons people stay in difficult relationships. You may feel complexly tied to your partner, perhaps by your long history together, financial or physical dependency, or a desire to maintain family stability for your children. The idea of walking away can feel intimidating and disorienting, especially if you have devoted much of your energy to raising kids. Perhaps you haven't worked for a while and worry about how you will support yourself. Or you may be in a caregiving role to your partner and feel reluctant to leave her/him without your help. Even if you are emotionally prepared to end the relationship, those considerations may lead you to remain with your partner or remain temporarily until you feel the time is more appropriate for leaving.

Whatever your reasons are for staying and for however long, there are things you can do to reduce conflict and improve things for yourself. These are things that help in any relationship but can be particularly effective in dealing with a narcissist.

1. Adjust Your Expectations

Be realistic. Narcissists are very unlikely to change and will only do so if they are motivated *for themselves*. The only person you can change is you, and the only thing you can change in the relationship is how you act and respond. Accept that you can't change your partner. Accept that you won't get certain needs met in the relationship.

2. Align Your Needs with Your Partner's

As you are well aware of by now, one way or another, narcissists will always put their needs before yours. If you can find ways to align your needs with your partner's, you'll function better and improve how you both feel. For example, if you want your partner to help more with the kids, find something s/he likes to do that s/he can do with them. This allows her/him to feel competent and like a good parent while the kids get positive time with her/him and you get a break.

3. Help Your Partner Feel Successful

We all want to feel successful in what we do, and this is particularly true of narcissists. Try to find ways you can support your partner in things that matter to her/him. Focus on what s/he does well rather than on her/his mistakes or flaws.

4. Acknowledge Your Partner's Strengths

Underneath the bluster and games, your partner above all wants to feel good about her-/himself. Try to find things about her/him that are genuine strengths that you can sincerely acknowledge and reinforce. Be specific and positive without false praise. If, for example, s/he takes pride as a cook, tell your partner when s/he makes things you like or when other people enjoy her/his cooking. If s/he is good at managing the household or finances, tell her/him that you appreciate it.

5. Try Not to Be Defensive

This is difficult, especially since you probably feel routinely mistreated and the narcissist may be pulling very ingrained triggers in you. But defensiveness with a narcissist will simply makes things worse for you. S/he will either feel pleasure from it and goad or punish you more, or will react with even fiercer defensiveness. As long as you feel you need to prove or explain something about yourself to the narcissist, you are opening yourself up to attack. *A narcissist does not care* about your feelings or reasons. Being self-aware and feeling confident in yourself is the best way to avoid reacting defensively.

6. Work on Yourself

As someone involved with a narcissist, particularly if it's a long-term relationship, you have probably deferred interests or goals for yourself. Try to reconnect with those parts of you. Take classes, go to therapy, get in shape, pursue hobbies—whatever makes you feel fulfilled.

7. Build in Happiness

Try to build as much happiness into your life as you can. Spend time doing things that are meaningful and enjoyable for you. If some of those things can include your partner, great. But if they don't, that's okay, too.

8. Connect with People

Find ways to fulfill your interpersonal needs outside the relationship. Spend time with people you care about, such as friends and your kids/grandkids. If that means leaving your partner at home, so be it.

9. Reassure Your Partner

Making changes, whether or not they directly affect your relationship, can be disorienting and even threatening, especially to the insecure narcissist. Reassure your partner (in whatever way works best) that the changes you are making are not a threat to your relationship but in fact are things you hope will make you both happy.

10. Plan for the Future

We all need to feel a sense of hope and purpose about the future. Think about your future. Make plans to do things that matter to you, with or without your partner.

Remember that there are ways to do the things on this list that do not involve manipulating, lying, or giving up on yourself. You—and your partner—will know when you are insincere.

LEAVING YOUR PARTNER

Breaking up is rarely easy. If your narcissistic partner leaves you, it can feel devastating. Especially if you have codependent issues (see Chapter 13), you may feel that you've lost a part of yourself you can't live without. However, if you do the leaving, even if you feel emotionally prepared or desperate to get out, you need to think it through and plan carefully before you take action.

As we have discussed, the narcissistic partner/spouse is controlling, hyperdefensive, unforgiving, and often spiteful and vindictive. Rejection is painful for all of us, but for the narcissist it is a searing injury that is likely to elicit harsh backlash. You may get lucky and have a relatively smooth break, but you should assume you won't and plan accordingly. Careful preparation is especially important if you are married and/or have kids together. Here are steps to take *before* discussing separation or divorce with your partner:

1. Consider Your Partner's Past Behavior

Look at your partner's history to predict likely reactions now. Think about how your partner has reacted before to previous rejection, breakups, and/ or feelings of being mistreated by you or others. Is s/he the type to shrink away, lash out, conduct a smear campaign, or grab your assets? Do not make the mistake of assuming you will be the exception or that your partner will honor your history together in any way.

2. Resist Backsliding

Mentally prepare yourself for the possibility that your partner will attempt to convince you to stay through desperate pleas, promises of reform, threats, guilt trips, or other forms of manipulation. Coach yourself in advance for these situations and have a rehearsed response that you can use under pressure and self-doubt. You may want to write down all your reasons for leaving and have the list to remind yourself and/or share your situation with a friend who can support you by being a voice of reason when you need it.

3. Control Your Assets

Your partner may attempt to seize or even destroy your things or things you share, including money, belongings, property, investments, animal companions, and the kids. Make sure you know what you have together and where it is (such as bank accounts and credit cards) and take steps to secure and protect what is yours. Don't underestimate your narcissistic partner's potential for ruthless self-interest and retaliatory harm.

4. Choose an Attorney Who Knows Narcissism

It is crucial to find an attorney who understands the narcissistic personality and has experience handling high-conflict divorce. A lawyer who is unaware of the realities of NPD is apt to make strategic mistakes that can have disastrous consequences for you and your kids. Such a lawyer may misinterpret or fail to recognize your partner's manipulations and out of ignorance perhaps even judge and undermine you. These days there are more and more lawyers familiar with narcissism and how to manage it in court. Consult with them before hiring to make sure they really do understand NPD and narcissistic divorce issues relevant to you, such as child custody and parental alienation.

5. Avoid Narcissistic Attorneys

When looking for legal representation, also keep in mind that lawyers too can be narcissistic or have full-blown NPD and that the profession often attracts and rewards such personalities. Pay attention to red flags such as poor listening, bragging, and grand promises. Be skeptical of lawyers who spend more time billing you than working on your behalf.

6. Document Abuse

Document agreements you make with your partner, your correspondences, and evidence of your partner's abuses. Take screen shots and photos, save texts and messages, and tell trusted family or friends about abusive incidents, so you have evidence to use in court and/or with the police if you need it.

7. Don't Let Guilt Dictate Your Decisions

Especially if your partner uses passive-aggressive forms of manipulation, s/he may attempt to use guilt to get you to agree to unreasonable terms when you are dividing your assets and determining child custody. Your partner may try to guilt you into accepting inequitable arrangements or giving away what is rightfully yours.

8. Have a Place to Go

Even if you plan to keep your home, you should be prepared to leave if the narcissist refuses to go or gets violent. Have a place you can go with your children, animals, and important belongings, including family heirlooms. Don't underestimate what the narcissist is capable of. In extreme cases, narcissists seize assets, destroy property, and take and/or even harm kids and pets.

9. Limit Your Partner's Access

Limit your partner's access to you and perhaps to your kids and pets. That may mean changing locks, blocking calls and texts, adjusting social media privacy settings, and the like. If the narcissist is threatening you, stalking, and/or entering your home or car without permission, it may be necessary to take out a restraining order, install an alarm system, inform your children's school about your custody arrangement, and/or relocate.

10. Have a Support Team

If only for emotional support, you need people you can confide in and who have your back. For more complicated breakups, you may need help with the kids, a place to stay, a place to store your things, financial assistance, and witnesses. Remember to reach out to people who know the realities of what you're dealing with. People who don't, even if they mean well, can make things worse, not better.

11. Minimize Conflict

Even if you taste bile at the thought of your partner, try to rise above and reduce conflict with him or her as much as possible. Since the narcissistic personality is reactive, unreasonable, and prone to rage, provoking him/her will only escalate harm to yourself.

12. Think Before You Act

Resist the impulse to react or jump to decisions. It may be tempting to give up things like belongings, assets, or even custody rights so you can end the unpleasantness now, but you and your kids will have to live with those choices perhaps for the rest of your lives. Instead give yourself time to think things through, consider the long-term picture, and consult with people you trust before taking any important steps in the separation/divorce process.

 PIT BULL LAWYER

When Sally decided to leave her thirty-five-year marriage, she hired a lawyer who had a reputation for being a "pit bull." "I needed someone to stand up to my rich husband and his lawyers, and I thought this guy would fight for me," she said. Not wanting to rock the boat and believing it was the price she had to pay for having an aggressive lawyer, Sally ignored warning signs about him such as not taking her calls and raising his fees when he learned she had personal savings. "I realized too late that yet another narcissist had walked into my life," she said. "I used all my savings to pay him and ended up with nothing in the divorce." ‹‹

fifteen

Parenting with a Narcissist

WITH A NARCISSISTIC PARENT, YOUR CHILDREN ARE AT RISK FOR LAST-ing emotional and physiological trauma. As the healthier parent, you can best support your children by honoring and validating them for who they are—not who the other parent says they are or insists they be. This is import-ant in any family, but it requires conscious attention and emphasis in the nar-cissistic family because of the narcissistic parent's invalidating influence. Such parents lack foundational stability and suffer from compulsive shame that drives them in a vicious cycle of attention-seeking and self-aggrandizement. Internally they are up or down depending on how well or how poorly their defensive compensations are serving them. In the process, they inevitably send invalidating messages to their children, intended or not. The invalidation may be direct, in the form of ignoring or scapegoating, or it may appear "pos-itive" in the form of idealized projection. But whether a child is ignored, criti-cized, or idealized, who they are is sacrificed in the narcissist's hall of mirrors. Tragically, narcissistic parents typically treat their children to the invalidating objectification that triggered their own disorder, perpetuating the trauma.

PROTECTING YOUR CHILDREN
FROM YOUR NARCISSISTIC SPOUSE

As the parent fortified with awareness of the dysfunction and its potential for harm, you have the opportunity to help scaffold your kids so they can weather the storms with strong self-esteem and coping skills. Many of us face difficulties in childhood, and your children can overcome theirs with support to counterbalance the narcissistic messages.

Stop Blaming Yourself

To start, let go of self-blame and regret. These are natural feelings once you come to understand the true nature of your narcissistic partner/spouse. But we all make mistakes in love and life. Chances are, when you got involved with your partner, you had no idea what you were getting into. Narcissists are skilled at drawing people in and hiding their selfishness, for a while. Or perhaps you believed you could fix or heal the narcissist, not understanding that her/his personality disorder was ingrained in early life and that changing is a very difficult process s/he has to do her-/himself. Possibly you were raised in a narcissistic or otherwise dysfunctional home yourself and were repeating the pattern as an adult, unaware that there were (and still are) better kinds of relationships available to you, or believing you were not worthy of them.

You did your best with the tools available to you. Whatever the reason you involved yourself with a narcissistic partner, wasting energy on guilt and regret will only make things harder for you and your kids.

WAYS TO SUPPORT YOUR CHILDREN

As the healthier adult in the family, you can do a lot to support your kids. You can't change the fact that their other parent is narcissistic. But you can improve the situation for your children and help them develop resilience and coping strategies. In addition to the following things you can do, your kids may benefit from seeing a counselor who understands narcissistic family dynamics (see Chapter 19).

1. Validate Their Feelings

A crucial thing to do for your kids is to validate their feelings. You may be tempted to try to shield yourself and/or them by denying their confusion and pain. But denying a child's rightful feelings protects no one. It only furthers the abuse and trauma, and it will destroy your child's trust in you.

Since the narcissistic parent routinely invalidates others through various means, such as dismissal, criticism, and mockery, your kids are especially in need of acknowledgment that their feelings are real and worthy of respect.

It is vital to validate that their feelings of hurt and anger are justified, particularly for the child who is scapegoated the most. They need to know that they don't deserve the treatment they are getting and the situation is not their fault or responsibility. Invalidation can happen in many ways, but the essential experience is to not be acknowledged, accepted, and/or respected for who we are, which includes our thoughts and emotions, our needs and curiosities, our likes and dislikes, and our self-expressions. The more you can do to support them and buffer them from harm, the better.

2. Give Credit Where Credit Is Due

Invalidation also happens when we do not receive appropriate acknowledgment for our accomplishments. Narcissists resent credit accorded to others and feel they are entitled to credit even when it is not earned, often distorting the truth or blatantly lying to get it. Narcissistic parents often refuse to admit a child's abilities or achievements or claim credit that rightfully belongs to that child. For example, a father may diminish and take credit for his child's athletic achievements by saying the child inherited abilities from him, learned skills from him, and/or benefited from help he paid for. Make sure to acknowledge your children's successes, even and especially when their other parent does not. If that parent is combative, it may be safer to express the acknowledgment privately.

3. Help Them Resist Blaming Themselves

Narcissists compulsively blame others, including for their own bad behavior. If narcissists throw a temper tantrum, they will always say someone or something else drove them to it. If they experience disappointment or hardship, someone else must be responsible. For narcissists, blaming others, particularly a scapegoated child, is as natural and necessary as breathing. Helping your children understand that their narcissistic parent's blame is unfounded and unfair is critical to their sense of an accurate reality. Seeing that they are not to blame will also relieve your kids of a heavy burden that should not be theirs to carry.

4. Tell the Truth

The fact about truth is that *you* need to see and acknowledge it yourself before you can help your kids do the same. Telling the truth is very tricky terrain in the narcissistic family—both dangerous and essential for those trying to cope with the narcissist's destructive influence. Narcissists have pathologically distorted ideas about themselves and those around them and are extremely invested in defending their distortions and compelling others to support them. Telling your kids that their father or mother is a narcissist or has a personality disorder and giving them details can potentially backfire badly if they tell your partner what you said.

Children are able to handle different levels of information depending on their age and maturity level. You have to use your best judgment about when and how much of the reality about your narcissistic spouse and family life to share with your children. You may want to reserve using the term *narcissist*, for example, until your child is a teenager or older. For younger children, explaining that their mother or father is very sensitive to criticism or perceived rejection and overreacts is an approach you could take. Emphasize that your narcissistic spouse's anger is extreme and not your child's fault or responsibility.

Children often perceive more than adults realize they do, and chances are they have insight into their narcissistic parent already. Kids are usually your best guide to what they are ready to hear. Waiting until your child asks about something often is the right way to introduce information. How you speak with your children will evolve naturally over time as they come to understand the family dynamics better.

5. Don't Demonize Your Narcissistic Spouse

Be careful not to demonize your spouse (even if s/he acts like a demon), as this can lead to confusion and ambivalence in your kids who, especially when young, will in most cases love and seek approval from their other parent no matter how badly s/he behaves. Tempering your own feelings about your spouse, who may be highly abusive, can feel next to impossible. But resisting your desire to cut loose with your own hurt, resentment, and anger is imperative in maintaining communication and trust with your kids, who are stuck in the middle. As your kids get older, you will be able to talk about things more openly and perhaps share information and resources with them about narcissistic personality disorder.

6. Avoid "Tough Love"

With exceptions, so-called tough love is not an effective parenting style, especially with children in a narcissistic home. With a narcissistic parent, they have endured the harshest of circumstances—an atmosphere of constant judgment and negation of self. Your children have already had it quite tough indeed, even if they are outwardly "spoiled." Although letting natural consequences play out is often useful, excessive pressure, control, or criticism is likely to trigger and alienate your children and add to their suffering.

7. Help Them Develop Resilience

Our most important job as parents is to foster resilience in our children so they can face life's challenges on their own two stable feet. This is particularly true for children in a narcissistic family. The best thing you can do for them is to model and nurture resilience by providing

- unconditional love (of which their other parent is incapable);
- acceptance, respect, and support for their individuality;
- an empathetic response to others;
- encouragement of hard work and accomplishments, without false praise;
- appropriate limits and flexibility; and
- reinforcement of confidence in and respect for their own feelings and instincts.

8. Don't Take Their Anger Personally

It's not fair, but your kids may at times vent their worst frustrations at you. This is because they cannot be honest with their narcissistic parent, and they trust you enough to act out and show their real feelings. They need to exorcise the pain and trauma they are dealing with, and although it is a double bind for you as someone who already may be taking the brunt of the narcissist's rages and manipulations, you will be called upon to rise above the crazy and be strong for your children. This does not mean, however, that you should put up with abuse from your kids. Your steady devotion and nondefensiveness is a lifeline for your children, but you also need to model self-respect, strength, and proper boundaries.

9. Talk about Their Rights

Even if your kids ostensibly know what fairness and human rights should be, they will carry confusion and doubt from having had their own basic rights undermined by their narcissistic parent in direct and indirect ways.

Remember your bill of rights from Chapter 1. You may want to share and discuss those rights with your children. Here is a modified version you can share with younger kids:

- **You can think your own thoughts.** You don't have to agree with others or have them agree with you. You don't have to share your thoughts if you don't want to.
- **You can feel your own feelings.** Feelings are an important part of being alive. Feelings are not bad or good; they just are. You don't have to act on your feelings, but you can if you think it matters. You don't have to feel what others feel or share your feelings if you don't want to.
- **Someone else's feelings and actions are their own, and you are not responsible for them.** You are responsible for your own feelings and actions, not anyone else's. You can't make someone feel or do things.
- **You have the right to love or not love.** Love is a feeling that can't be forced. Love is a good thing, and how you show it is up to you. Everyone shows their love in different ways.
- **If people love you, they do not ask you to change who you are.** You are lovable as you are. You don't have to change or be a certain way for anyone.
- **It's okay to be different.** Your job is to be yourself. Do your own best.
- **Love is what we do, not just what we say.** If someone says one thing but does something different, which thing matters more?
- **You are allowed to say what you think and feel.** You have the right to express yourself. You should try not to hurt people, but you can't control how other people feel or what they think about your feelings.
- **Each person is important in her or his own way.** We all have a place. We all matter. We all have strengths and weaknesses. No one is better or worse than anyone else, just different.
- **It's what's inside that counts.** Sometimes people focus on outside appearances, but what is inside each of us matters much more.

WAYS TO HELP YOUR CHILDREN COPE WITH FAMILY ROLES

In Chapters 8 and 17, we examine the roles that children commonly play in narcissistic families: golden child, hero, scapegoat, lost child, and mascot. These roles are dictated by the primary narcissist in the family and also reflect ways the children respond to their environment and attempt to deal with it. Children may play some or all of these roles at different times, especially if the family is small or if circumstances change. Sometimes kids play different roles with different parents. But often a child in a narcissistic family has one primary role. We revisit the roles here to address how you can help support children dealing with the particular burdens of each one. These are guidelines to help your kids break out of destructive patterns. It can also be very helpful to find a therapist for them with a good understanding of narcissistic family dynamics and trauma.

Help for the Golden Child

In the narcissistic family, the golden child is most enmeshed with the narcissistic parent, treated with privilege and favoritism while also experiencing entrapment. Just as the scapegoat serves as a projection of the narcissistic parent's hated and disowned self, the golden child functions as an extension of the narcissist's ideal self. Although this position in the family may appear "golden," the reality is that children in this role are pushed to sacrifice their authentic self for a false one dictated by their parents. Because such children receive attention and praise for things that may or may not reflect their actual interests, abilities, or achievements, they experience a dislocating sense of underlying effacement beneath their exaggerated importance. They often work to present well and excel and may become perfectionist to maintain their privileged status, but they struggle with self-doubt and cognitive dissonance arising from differences in how they are treated in their family versus in the world outside it.

Typically overindulged and spared criticism and accountability for their behavior, golden children can become self-centered and arrogant. Of all the roles, golden children may be most at risk for adopting the parent's narcissistic traits and perpetuating the generational trauma. Children who internalize the narcissistic parent's identity become bullies at home and school and grow into cruel and entitled adults who bury their fears and reassure themselves by aligning with forms of authority that reinforce their privilege. But the golden child may avoid this fate if shown enough care and empathy by a more functional parent or other adult. If such children are able to gain perspective outside the family and recognize the narcissist's treatment as the abuse it really is, they may be able to reconnect with their needs, accept responsibility for their actions, and build compassion for the inner self as well as for others. Engaging with their feelings, withholding judgment, practicing empathy, and building emotional literacy and authentic connections with others are roads to healing.

Here are ways to help golden children:

1. Model and reinforce an empathic response to people, animals, news stories, and so on.
2. Share and discuss books about perspectives and experiences different from their own to help them build awareness and empathy.
3. Encourage them to consider the points of view of other family members, in particular, the scapegoat.
4. Encourage them to explore genuine interests and pursuits other than what they have been rewarded for by the narcissistic parent.
5. Reinforce their hard work rather than innate ability or specific kinds of achievement.
6. Talk about black-and-white thinking and encourage a more complex perspective of people and relationships.
7. Model and discuss healthy physical and emotional boundaries.
8. Volunteer with them to help people or animals in need.

Help for the Hero/Scapegoat

Children in the role of hero may receive attention and praise for their strength, leadership, and achievements in and outside the family, but they carry a heavy burden. Although they often appear highly capable and may work hard to please and appease, they are after all still children who need and often crave caretaking but feel they have no choice but to be strong in the chaotic environment of home. Often the firstborn, heroes respond to their parents' dysfunction by picking up the slack around the house and in many cases distinguishing themselves at school and/or other areas of life. They may take on domestic responsibilities, such as cleaning, cooking, and looking after siblings, while also emotionally caretaking one or both parents. Their caretaking may include playing confidant, therapist, or surrogate spouse.

The hero role is different in the narcissistic family than in other kinds of dysfunctional families. Because the narcissistic parent habitually projects and engulfs, the golden child occupies the primary favored role. There may be no classic "hero" child in the narcissistic family, or there may be a child who functions in many ways as a hyperresponsible and/or caretaking hero but also experiences scapegoating. This **hero/scapegoat** does emotional and physical caretaking of family members that may include defending an abused enabling parent or siblings from the narcissist. Such a child may be scapegoated as a result of standing up to the narcissist, or s/he may be a scapegoated child who stands up out of concern for other abused family members. Often both dynamics are at work for a child in this position.

Children in a hero/scapegoat role find themselves working to keep the family functioning while being targeted by the primary narcissistic parent. They may feel a sense of pride and agency because of the help they provide but at the same time experience feelings of anguish and powerlessness against the narcissist's cruel domination. Their wish to rescue their enabling parent may be mixed with a feeling of betrayal at that parent's inability or unwillingness to support them. Not understanding the entrenched nature of their narcissistic parent's condition, they also may try to help her/him despite being that parent's punching bag.

Children in this position struggle with anger and despair over injustices they cannot put right and people they cannot rescue, most pointedly themselves. Their feelings of competency can help them see through the family dysfunction and fight against assaults to their self-esteem, but as scapegoats they internalize blame, defer their needs, and suffer with symptoms of CPTSD that can extend long into adulthood. Feeling needed but also exploited and abused, they swing between over- and underestimating their ability to influence others and effect change. In many ways they experience the worst of both roles—the scapegoat's victimization and the hero's overresponsibility. See "Help for the Scapegoat," next, for ways to support this child.

Help for the Scapegoat

The scapegoat child bears the blame for family misfortune and the negative actions of other family members. Having a designated scapegoat allows the parents to disown their shame and abuses and gives the family a target to rally around to disavow its problems. Typically labeled a screw-up or rebel, the scapegoat is often the most sensitive and/or independent-minded child who dares to question the parents and call out the family dysfunction. No matter what the scapegoat actually does, s/he rarely meets with approval and instead faces an ongoing smear campaign. The scapegoat may respond by acting out in anger and fulfilling the prescribed role of rebel/bad seed or becoming perfectionist to avoid attack while also pushing against the family's systemic lies. Such children are inevitably beaten down with negative messages that they can't help but internalize in the form of toxic guilt, shame, self-doubt, and self-destructive behavior. Having been routinely judged by their parents and possibly ganged up on by family members, they feel defensive, misunderstood, and painfully isolated. They are most likely to suffer with CPTSD, which can lead to a self-perpetuating cycle of health and financial problems in adulthood. But they also have both innate and learned strength, empathy, and awareness that give them great potential to heal and be healed if they can find perspective and support outside the family. Teachers, mentors, friends, animals, and other sources of validation and meaning, such as nature and art, can be life changing for scapegoats.

Here are ways to help scapegoat and hero/scapegoat children:

1. Listen to them and show respect for their feelings.
2. Acknowledge and validate their hurt and anger.
3. Empower them by encouraging a creative outlet, such as writing or playing an instrument.
4. Encourage connections for them with positive adults outside the family.
5. Help them accept mistakes and failures as learning experiences rather than character indictments.
6. Give them books with themes of scapegoating, bigotry, and justice to help them understand the larger picture.
7. Encourage them to pursue a sport or group membership so they experience being a valued member of a team.
8. Give them an outlet to work for justice in some way, such as by fighting climate change, helping marginalized people, or caring for animals.

Help for the Lost Child

The lost child is just that—overlooked and ignored. This child isn't invisible but may as well be to the parents. Often the third in larger families, the lost child is overshadowed by the idealized golden child and the negative attentions directed at the scapegoat. Feeling fundamentally burdensome in the chaotic family environment, the lost child denies her/his needs and avoids attention to keep from being targeted or placing further demands on the parents.

Lost children typically learn to disengage from their emotions, withdraw socially, and escape into an interior world of fantasy and distraction through solo activities such as reading, drawing, or gaming. Keeping a low profile helps the lost child avoid guilt and blame, but it also means sacrificing the self, including personal achievement and intimacy with others. Outside the family, the lost child plays the loner who aims high enough to avoid negative attention but low enough to remain unremarkable. As they get older and move into adulthood, lost children often feel like outsiders, find it difficult to identify what they want, and struggle with buried anger, emptiness, and depression. They need help to understand their feelings, resist self-effacement, reach out, and connect through meaningful work and relationships. Practicing self-awareness, identifying and expressing their needs, and forging closeness with others are important steps toward well-being.

Here are ways to help lost children:

1. Show interest in the things they like to do.
2. Reinforce them by being responsive when they attempt to connect or ask for help.
3. Build a quiet rapport with them that isn't too threatening in the family group but helps you stay connected.
4. Seek them out in ways that show you care without putting them on the spot in front of others.
5. Remind them that they are just as important in the family as anyone else and that you like it when they join in.
6. Encourage their strengths and interests.
7. Spend time alone together.
8. Check in with them about their feelings and help them articulate their needs.

Help for the Mascot

Often the youngest child, the mascot is the clowning distractor. Cute, funny, and/or entertaining, the mascot redirects the family from stress and discord with stories, jokes, hijinks, and other amusements. The mascot may be spared the worst abuse and at times treated with affection and indulgence. But that child is also infantilized, not taken seriously, and burdened with relieving the family of its sadness, while not being able to understand or solve the core problems.

Just as they temporarily divert the family from its dysfunction, mascots tend to dismiss and deny their own feelings, focus on others instead of themselves, and stay in motion to escape their confusion and pain. They often struggle to focus, grow up, and understand their needs, and they are at risk of escapist addictions and unhealthy enabling relationships. They can be quite empathetic and giving but find it difficult to feel worthy of respect and support. If they are successful people managers, like the hero they may fall into the trap of believing they are more powerful than they truly are and find it difficult to admit their needs and vulnerabilities. Resisting people-pleasing and developing more functional boundaries, self-awareness, and self-esteem beyond making others feel good is the mascot's path to fulfillment and healing.

Here are ways to help mascot children:

1. Validate them for personal interests and pursuits other than entertaining or managing others.
2. Help them identify and honor their needs and emotions.
3. Take them seriously and invite their opinions.
4. Be alert to problems at school and address them promptly.
5. Give them responsibilities so they can gain a sense of competency.
6. Encourage them to self-reflect and ask for what they want/need.
7. Encourage them to do solo activities or projects that build independence, self-awareness, and a sense of meaning.
8. Help them set and work toward long-term goals.

PROTECTING YOUR CHILDREN FROM CODEPENDENCY

Just as children need help to steer away from adopting narcissistic behaviors, they also need help to navigate away from codependent behaviors that have been modeled for them. Actively supporting them is important, but they also need you to show them that you respect and value yourself. To be able to do that, they need you to model healthier patterns in your life and relationships. Even if you are not prepared to leave your narcissistic partner, you can do many things to change your own behavior and improve things for yourself and your kids.

Your kids need you to show them that you:
1. Are willing to acknowledge reality
2. Understand and respect your own feelings
3. Take responsibility for yourself
4. Do not need to control things to feel okay
5. Accept your mistakes and weaknesses without blame or shame
6. Have your own opinions and interests
7. Have fulfilling relationships outside your family
8. Are not afraid of being alone
9. Do not value others over yourself
10. Will say no and follow through on it

Just by reading this book, you have taken a big step toward breaking your denial, identifying and understanding what you're dealing with, and making changes to help yourself and your children. The stronger and more aware you become, the better parent you will be. As you work to improve your situation and gain strategies for coping and healing, you are improving things for all of you. We explore more specific strategies in Part 6.

PARALLEL PARENTING WITH A NARCISSIST EX

Parenting is arguably the hardest work one can do in life, even with a loving and compatible partner. Coparenting with a narcissist ex is exponentially more difficult: draining, disorienting, divisive, and at times cause for feelings of black anger and despair.

Your Narcissist Ex Doesn't Love Your Kids the Way You Do

It is painful, perhaps incomprehensible, but your narcissistic ex will never love your children the way you do. On some level you already know this, even if you still struggle to accept the reality of it. In the extreme case, s/he may be flatly incapable of caring about them at all, instead using them as targets of sadistic and violent abuse. Even in less malignant circumstances, s/he will see them as extensions of her-/himself to be controlled and exploited.

Making matters worse, your narcissist ex's main objective may be to hurt *you*, regardless of how it harms your kids.

If you did the leaving, the rejected narcissist is likely to hold a profound long-term grudge, seeking to punish you for triggering her/his narcissist injury. If s/he left you, you are still fair game for propaganda and persecution. Whoever initiated the breakup, the narcissist is likely to use every opportunity to bolster her-/himself at your expense. S/he may insult and demean you in front of your children; engage in a smear campaign behind your back to your kids, extended family, and social circle; and undermine your efforts to communicate as a coparent.

KING OF THE CASTLE

As Iris was picking up her kids from her ex-husband's house, she noticed her son wasn't wearing shoes and asked him to go back in for them. When he hesitated and said they were "gone," she pressed him for an explanation until his older sister said, "Dad threw them out because he wore them in the house and we're not supposed to." Iris asked, "Why would he throw them out?!" Her daughter replied that their father had separate rules for them and rules for himself. She said, "He says the house is his castle and he gets to wear shoes and sit on the furniture and we don't." ‹‹

Forget Coparenting and Accept Parallel Parenting

Before young children develop the ability to play together cooperatively, they will parallel play with the same toys or games near each other but separately. Narcissists never learn truly cooperative play, and the same goes for their ability to parent. Fairness and teamwork are outside their playbook. Rather than working with you in your children's best interests, your ex will vie for your children's attention and adoration, often at your expense, using whatever tools are at hand, such as gifts, permissiveness, and false promises. Your ex may also bail out on parenting if/when it loses value (i.e., becomes costly, taxing, boring, irritating).

Sharing custody of your children with your narcissistic ex, you need to toss out the normal rules of engagement, including expectations of cooperation, shared values and goals, and healthy communication. As painful as this is about the other parent of your children, you need to accept reality and embrace minimalist parallel parenting. This means limiting your interactions with your ex to gain control, avoid conflict, and reduce your vulnerability to manipulation. This is important for both you and your kids.

Parallel Parenting Do List

1. Do establish a regular visitation schedule and stick to it.
2. Do limit contact/communication with your ex to absolute essentials.
3. Do keep clear and strict boundaries with your ex.
4. Do withhold your true feelings/thoughts from your ex.
5. Do ignore your ex's antagonisms, whether passive-aggressive or overtly aggressive.
6. Do let natural consequences play out for your ex.
7. Do take the high road and avoid getting into petty disputes with your ex.
8. Do accept that you cannot control your ex's parenting, even if it sucks.
9. Do have faith in your own parenting (one attuned good parent is more powerful than several bad parents/stepparents—really).
10. Do be as honest as you can (age appropriately) with your kids about your family situation.
11. Do accept parenting help from supportive family/friends.
12. Do try to limit communication, such as texting, between your kids and their other parent when they are with you.

Parallel Parenting Don't List

1. Don't argue with your ex.
2. Don't make yourself vulnerable to your ex.
3. Don't share personal information with your ex.
4. Don't react to your ex's barbs or criticisms.
5. Don't take your ex's version of events, particularly regarding your kids, at face value.
6. Don't internalize your ex's projections.
7. Don't try to explain your concerns about your kids to your ex.
8. Don't ever criticize your kids to your ex, as s/he will use it against them/you.
9. Don't engage emotionally with your ex. Go gray rock: boring, flat, monotonous.

10. Don't blame yourself for your ex's behavior.
11. Don't allow your ex to violate boundaries you've established.
12. Don't forget that although your ex may be a jerk, the silver lining of your relationship is your kids.

Document, Document, Document

Finally, you need to be prepared to defend yourself and your children with legal protections and documentation of the narcissist's abuses. Narcissists see themselves as above rules and laws and do not hesitate to manipulate them for their gain. They may violate parenting plans, break agreements, ignore appointments and schedules, call or text at all hours, show up unannounced, engage in stalking, verbally and perhaps physically assault you and your kids, and the list goes on. You may need to take steps to limit the narcissist's access to you and your children and carefully and consistently document her/his violations, have witnesses, and assume that s/he may be recording everything you say and do.

PARENTAL ALIENATION AND PARENTAL ALIENATION SYNDROME

Parental alienation occurs when one parent influences a child to distrust, disrespect, and/or reject the other parent. Because of their compulsive splitting (viewing people as all good or all bad), need to be right and superior, desire for control, and low to absent concern for the well-being of family members, parents with NPD are more likely than most to attempt to weaken a partner's or ex's relationships with their children, particularly during a divorce and/or custody dispute. The narcissistic parent's alienating influence may consist of criticisms that undermine respect and trust, or it may take extreme form as parental alienation syndrome (PAS), in which the child is brainwashed to the point that s/he becomes a participant in the denigration and rejection of the targeted parent. Men and woman alike may engage in and suffer from parental alienation.

Some degree of parental alienation is common in narcissistic families. As we have discussed, narcissistic parents attempt to disrupt bonds between other members of the family through smear campaigns, triangulation, and other manipulations. Separation and divorce from a narcissistic partner doesn't necessarily but can escalate such behavior. Depending on the particular personalities and dynamics of the family, children may be relatively immune to such influence, or they may become so enmeshed with the antagonistic narcissistic parent that they adopt that parent's language and behavior, become distrustful of the targeted parent, and perhaps refuse contact with the alienated parent.

Estrangement versus Alienation

Estrangement between a parent and child is different from alienation. Estrangement can occur when a parent chooses not to communicate with a child or have contact, or if a child rightfully pulls away from an abusive parent. For example, an older child may choose not to see a verbally or physically assaultive parent or one with addictions or other problems that make contact unmanageable. Alienation, on the other hand, is its own form of abuse that happens when one parent undermines a child's relationship with a targeted parent. The influence of an alienating parent can range from mild to severe. A parent may disparage an ex out of anger and lack of self-control, or in extreme cases, a parent may conduct a deliberate campaign to disrupt or destroy a child's relationship with a targeted parent.

A child driven into a state of unwarranted parental alienation may experience deep and potentially lasting damage. For the alienated healthier parent in this scenario, the reality is heartbreaking, but it is by no means reason to give up hope of reconnecting and repairing the rupture. If you are seeing signs of alienation in a child, seek therapeutic support and legal counsel from professionals knowledgeable about the issue.[1]

PART 5

CHILDREN OF NARCISSISTS

The Under- and Overparented Child

F OR CHILDREN IN THE DYSFUNCTIONAL NARCISSISTIC HOME, LIFE IS CHAR-
acterized by imbalance and disparity. Adults' needs overshadow children's. Siblings compete, often brutally, for inadequate resources. Couples
are combative or estranged. Outsiders fail to see anything wrong, or
recognize the dysfunction but don't know how to help. Parents flip-flop
between overindulging and neglecting their kids. One child is elevated,
while another is denigrated. One child is given adult responsibilities,
while another is infantilized. Just as the parents swing emotionally from
inflation to deflation, children are treated to extremes of idealization and
rejection, overdependency and abandonment.

Unlike emotionally mature and stable parents whose priority is to meet
their children's needs, support their healthy development, and respect and
nurture their individual identity, narcissistic parents put their own needs
first and objectify their kids in service of those needs. Whether they treat
them as trophies, competitors, mini-me projections, sacrificial lambs, inden-
tured servants, court jesters, or stray dogs, narcissistically disordered parents
compulsively negate and dehumanize their kids. Such children experience a
disrupted childhood and heavy burdens that they struggle to bear long into
their adult lives. Interactions among family members are dictated by the lies
the parents tell, and the children believe the lies about themselves and one
another to a lesser or greater extent depending on their ability to distance
themselves from the family and think independently.

Living with a narcissist is traumatic for other adults, but children are most vulnerable to harm because they are

- dependent on their parents for survival,
- dependent on their parents for validation and development of self,
- impressionable and susceptible to their parents' opinions, and
- easy and manipulatable targets.

IDEALIZATION AND DEVALUATION

Narcissistic parents fail to see themselves or their children in a realistic light. Just as they vacillate between their own self-aggrandizement and shame, they treat their children to ongoing patterns of overvaluation, undervaluation, or fluctuation between the two extremes. Typically one child is routinely idealized in the role of golden child and another is scapegoated, but at any given time *any child in the family may be targeted with exaggerated favor or disfavor.* In a home with one child, that child will probably be primarily targeted as a scapegoat or elevated as a golden child, but also will experience a roller coaster of idealizing and devaluing treatment.

Children perpetually faced with highs and lows of favoritism and invalidation or who routinely witness their siblings treated to such extremes[1] experience sustained trauma. Never safe, they are constantly working to win approval and avoid being targeted. Trapped on the family stage, they learn to perform in whatever roles are available to them with the limited tools they may have. Who they are is sacrificed in the family hierarchy, which is dictated by the parents and ruled on high by the dominant narcissist. Read more about idealizing, scapegoating, and coping with child roles in Chapters 8, 15, and 17.

PARENTIFICATION: THE UPSIDE-DOWN CHILD-PARENT RELATIONSHIP

Consistent, appropriate caretaking and unconditional love are beyond the narcissist's scope. Rather than seeing those things as their responsibilities and privileges as a parent, narcissists expect such treatment from their kids, often turning the adult-child relationship upside down.

In the narcissistic home, it is common for the parents to parentify one or more of their children, expecting them to meet their emotional and sometimes physical needs and fulfill roles beyond their maturity level or rightful responsibility. The parentified child may be treated as best friend, counselor, surrogate spouse, or a combination of those roles. That child also may be burdened with excessive chores, caretaking siblings, managing finances, or earning money for the household.

Parentified children may feel flattered to be given adult responsibilities and honored to play the role of "special helper." It may feel as though they are getting attention and validation from their parent that they can't get any other way. But parentification is an extreme violation of boundaries. Parentified children are used at their own expense to meet the needs of the person whose job it is to meet theirs. They experience a truncated childhood if one at all. As they mature, such children are likely to struggle with perfectionism and confusion about boundaries, fall into caretaking roles, and believe they can only gain love and approval by working for it.

NEGLECT

Narcissistic abuse is typically understood as a set of overbearing behaviors stemming from narcissists' outsize self-importance and lack of empathy. Narcissists dominate family members with their excessive neediness, selfish demands, antagonism, hypersensitivity, and unrealistic expectations. But neglect, both physical and emotional, also is a defining feature of narcissistic homes, with devastating impact.

As opposed to outright abuse, neglect is the *absence* of support and therefore can be difficult to identify, even and especially for the person neglected, particularly a child. Child Welfare Information Gateway (CWIG) identifies neglect as the most common form of child abuse and sites data showing that chronically neglected children have "more severe cognitive and academic deficits [and] social withdrawal" than children abused in other ways. CWIG defines four primary types of neglect (with some of my own additions here):

1. Physical neglect: failure to meet a child's basic survival needs for food, clothing, hygiene, and shelter; and failure to provide supervision and safe conditions

2. Medical neglect: failure to meet a child's health care needs
3. Educational neglect: failure to ensure a child receives an adequate education to think critically and function in society
4. Emotional neglect: failure to provide a child with attention, affection, empathy, and other forms of emotional nurturing[2]

All types of neglect can occur in a narcissistic family. Narcissists' self-focus and low to absent concern for others inevitably translate into negligent parenting. Although social pressures to fulfill parenting roles and provide the appearance of normalcy or even exceptionalism drive many narcissistic parents to meet their children's most obvious needs, frequently children in such homes receive sporadic and highly conditional care. An infection may go unnoticed until it is severe. An unsupervised child may get injured, in trouble with the police, or violated by an older child or adult. A habitually hungry child may look for steady meals at a neighbor's or friend's house. A child may be burdened with so much responsibility at home that s/he drops out of school. A serially ignored child may turn to drugs, self-harm, or unsafe sex to manage loneliness and depression.

Children in narcissistic families may also suffer with gaps and handicaps in their practical preparedness for life outside the family. They may lack knowledge of or experience with basic life skills because their parents are unable or unwilling to advise them or teach them how to do things. Even parentified "superkids" in such families, who appear precocious, usually have significant deficits that can make it difficult to function in adolescence and adulthood.

Learning Not to Need

Children from narcissistic homes learn early on *not to need*. Such children are taught through words and deeds, tones and silences that in the universe of home their parents' needs take precedence and their own are often cause for resentment and even punishment. Since we all need physical and emotional support at any age, but particularly when we are relatively helpless children with little knowledge of the world or power over our circumstances, such messages are devastating.

Children taught not to need look for ways to survive without their parents. They attempt to mask their vulnerabilities and bury their feelings, things that are ultimately impossible in the long run. Inevitably they feel shame about their normal needs and learn to fear and hate their own human vulnerability. Neglected children may appear unkempt, with unwashed hair and clothes, untreated illnesses and injuries, and malnourishment. But signs of neglect, particularly emotional neglect, are often behavioral and less obvious. Neglected children may display a range of symptoms, including

- flat affect,
- inattention,
- withdrawal/self-isolation,
- emotional reactivity,
- low self-esteem,
- proneness to guilt,
- unresponsiveness to pain,
- dissociation,
- difficulty communicating, and/or
- risk-taking.

Neglect is hard enough to endure for any child, but in the narcissistic home, it is often exacerbated by messages from impaired parents that they are perfect and their children are fortunate to get whatever they offer. Extremely narcissistic parents fundamentally feel they don't "owe" their children anything, and when they do things for their kids they typically expect something in return, such as profuse appreciation, compliance, or some form of service. For narcissists, relationships are transactional, and they expect to get more than they give.

Children quickly learn to rely on their more responsive parent to meet their day-to-day needs and to show gratitude for even the most basic gestures from their narcissistic parent. When both parents are narcissistic or otherwise impaired, children learn to manipulate to meet their needs, rely on siblings or other family members, and/or look outside the home.

Narcissistic parents, especially mothers, who derive a sense of identity and self-worth from the belief that they are wonderful parents often go to great lengths to appear to the outside world that they are exceptionally dedicated and caring. They may regard anything less than perfect performance and behavior from their children as a personal slight and a public embarrassment. To their social network, they may criticize, pathologize, and "disown" their scapegoated child as a disappointment, source of worry,

and/or troublemaker, garnering sympathy for their suffering, while holding up their golden child as a projection of their idealized self-beliefs and
evidence of their great parenting.

Children of narcissistic parents experience a cognitive dissonance, or
conflict between reality and what they are told is happening, about the
neglect in their home. They naturally feel empty, frightened, and angry
(unconsciously or consciously) about their parent's neglect but constantly
receive the message that the parent is above reproach. Narcissistic fathers
may be touted for being generous and dedicated providers while mothers
are loving and self-sacrificing caregivers. For children dealing with a very
different reality, the neglect becomes that much harder to recognize. They
must deny reality or blame themselves rather than admit that the family line
is a lie and the care they are getting is tragically deficient.

ENGULFMENT

In the narcissistic home, the flip side but not opposite of neglect is engulfment. Also referred to as *enmeshment,* engulfment is a common parenting
style of narcissists, particularly with golden children. Engulfment is, in
essence, parents' blurring boundaries between themselves and their child,
absorbing or subsuming the child's identity into their own and their own
into the child's. Narcissistic parents engulf their children fundamentally
because they lack a stable core identity and are looking to fill the void. And
who better to fill that emptiness than an impressionable, malleable child
under their control?

Healthy Childhood Individuation

It is normal to identify with our children and certainly for them to identify with us. That bond of identification and modeling between parent and
child is one of the pleasures of parenting and crucial for healthy childhood
development. Yet as with most things in life, there is a necessary balance
between parental involvement and the child's emerging individuality. Parenting is a continuous recalibration of that balance in the relationship as
the child increasingly forms and expresses an autonomous self and the
parents adjust their parenting style to match the child's changing needs.
Indeed, the adjustments between parents and children occur throughout

the relationship as long as both are alive. The secure and responsive parent
is attentive and flexible, involved and independent, nurturing the child's
evolving identity like a growing garden.

Disrupted Individuation

In contrast, engulfing parents do not recognize or respect their children's individual personhood. In the narcissistic family's upside-down parent-child
relationship, children are expected to serve and adjust to the narcissistic
parents' needs and reflect back the version of selfhood that those parents
wish to see, regardless of how true it feels to the children. A child's developmental need to individuate is ignored, and movements toward such development are met with forceful resistance. Qualities the parents value are
rewarded, and ones the parents dislike or are threatened by are discouraged
and suppressed through denial, criticism, shame, and/or punishment. The
engulfed child suffers profound boundary violations, including emotional,
psychological, physical, and sometimes sexual ones.

In relationship to their golden child, engulfing parents may

1. project their own hopes and dreams onto the child;
2. look for parenting from the child;
3. look for companionship and intimacy, sometimes sexual, from the
   child;
4. resent the child's steps toward independence;
5. infantilize the child to feel needed;
6. expect the child to adopt their beliefs and opinions;
7. expect agreement and acquiescence from the child;
8. be jealous of and interfere in the child's other relationships;
9. attempt to win over and "own" the child's friends; and/or
10. expect the child to prioritize them over all others.

Often children dealing with engulfing parents attempt to repress and
hide their genuine interests and inclinations in an effort to meet parents' expectations of who they should be. Such children typically learn to dissociate
from their "unacceptable" feelings. The engulfed child feels like an impostor, constantly reading the narcissistic parents' reactions and making adjustments to please the parents at the expense of authenticity. Below the surface,
such children may experience confusion, anxiety, inadequacy, guilt, shame,

resentment, anger, and feelings of entrapment. They may become adept at manipulating, people-pleasing, and/or lying—both to others and themselves.

Engulfment seems quite different from neglect on the surface, but boiled down, it resembles emotional neglect in that the child's personhood is ignored. In both situations, the needs of the narcissistic parents are foremost, and their child's authentic self is eclipsed. Such dynamics can persist in adulthood, with the engulfed adult child feeling overshadowed by the narcissistic parent's endless demands for attention and control.

INFANTILIZATION

In the narcissistic home, parents may infantilize their engulfed children, treating them as if they are much younger than their age. Parents infantilize their kids as a means of control, as a way to feel needed or superior, and because they do not recognize or respect their boundaries.

Parents infantilize children/adult children by

1. speaking for them,
2. deciding for them,
3. stepping in to handle things for them,
4. questioning their decisions,
5. judging/criticizing their choices,
6. offering unsolicited advice,
7. intruding in their relationships,
8. interfering at school or work,
9. restricting their freedoms, and/or
10. demanding compliance.

Infantilizing children/adult children undermines their confidence and keeps them insecure and dependent, enabling narcissistic parents to meet their own continuous need to feel needed, superior, and perhaps heroic to outsiders. Rather than helping their children build self-sufficiency, infantilizing parents attempt to keep their children in a state of self-doubt and helpless dependency. In extreme cases, infantilizing parents may dress and feed older children, do their homework, choose their friends and dates, choose their college or career, and otherwise attempt to manage the most basic parts of their lives well into adulthood. As adults, such children may continue to live at home and rely on their parents for companionship, caretaking, financial support, and other fundamental aspects of their survival. For such children, their codependent relationship is fraught with ambivalence, shame, fear, and anger.

OVERINDULGENCE

At first glance, overindulgent parenting can be mistaken for agreeability, generosity, even love. What child doesn't want more dessert, fewer chores, additional screen time, or the chance to stay up late? Such indulgences once in a while are fun, especially as a reward for hard work or a break from normal routines. But indulgence that is habitual rather than the exception has serious, even devastating consequences for kids.

Overindulgence as Neglect

As we have discussed, one of the most important things we do for our children is to set appropriate boundaries for them, which include both restrictions and freedoms/responsibilities. Overindulgence can be too much or too little of something and not saying no or yes when necessary. Children rely on adults to supervise their evolving capabilities, fostering their growth while providing healthy and safe conditions in which to experiment and learn. Children who are chronically overindulged are not healthy or safe. Their fundamental need for appropriate boundaries is neglected.

In some cases, it is the children who appear most indulged who are suffering the worst neglect. Their parents may lavish them with possessions and privileges such as toys, cars, credit cards, and admission into clubs and colleges while failing to supervise their day-to-day lives, show affection, spend time with them, or teach them life skills. Such children may be given excessive entitlements, bailed out of consequences, told they are better than their peers, and paraded as one more marker of their parents' superiority while being starved of genuine love and caretaking.

Wonky Boundaries

In narcissistic families, boundaries are often wildly askew. A defining characteristic of narcissistic parenting is a failure to set or respect children's necessary boundaries. As with other things in the family, limits and freedoms are determined not by the child's needs but instead by the parents'. A mother who refuses to let her child be held by anyone but herself prioritizes her own need for control and to feel needed over the baby's need to have contact with other people. Parents who don't watch over their toddler care more about their own agenda than the toddler's need for attentive supervision. A father who does his child's homework cares more about his child getting a good grade than the child's need to learn and take responsibility. Parents who don't supervise their teenager's activities at night are prioritizing their own plans or avoiding conflict over their child's safety.

Because of their extreme selfishness and lack of emotional intelligence and empathy, narcissistic parents fail to provide their children with age-appropriate boundaries, whether emotional, psychological, physical, or sexual. Such boundaries may be too strict, too lenient, or altogether absent because narcissistic parents objectify their children as means to their own ends. Often such parents themselves have been treated to similar negligence and abuse and are repeating harmful generational patterns.

Indulgent parenting is especially confusing for children because, on the surface, it can appear to be something desired. Often a narcissistic parent presents it as an act of "love" for which children should feel lucky. A father who plies his kids with junk food and ignores bedtime may win points as the "fun" parent, while avoiding the harder job of preparing healthy food and managing their need for sleep. A mother who oversees every aspect of her children's lives may appear caring and dedicated, while fulfilling her own desire for attention and control at the expense of their need for individuation.

Although children in these situations may regard such parenting as normal or even special, they inevitably feel unseen and unsafe. Consciously or unconsciously, they long for secure and appropriate boundaries that they see in other families, at school, and in books and on screen. These kids may react against or feel around for boundaries at home by acting out in extreme or rebellious ways, hoping to get responsive adult involvement. They may attempt to take on the job of boundary-setting for themselves and their siblings by becoming hyperresponsible. Or they may become passive and compliant, hoping their narcissistic parent will take care of them if they acquiesce to that parent's demands. However these children attempt to adapt to overindulgent parenting, they are likely to struggle with boundaries in their lives beyond their family of origin, not knowing where they and others begin and end.

THE FUN PARENT

Ben and his ex-wife shared custody of their son Henry. After staying with his mother, Henry would return to Ben's house tired, stressed out, and unwashed because his mother let him watch television after bedtime, ignore his homework, and skip showers. "She thought of herself as the 'fun parent,'" Ben said. "By the time she'd drop Henry off with me, he was a basket case—crabby from lack of sleep, dirty, and worried about his homework. I'd have to pick up the pieces and play the disciplinarian who made him do his work, bathe, and get to bed. Bringing it up with her just made things more combative between us, so I had to make the best of it until Henry got old enough to take better care of himself at her house. It was infuriating!" ⟨⟨

OVERPRAISING

As is the case with overindulgence, overvaluing a child for certain traits or achievements while ignoring or devaluing others can send harmful messages. Overpraising tends to normalize praise itself and can lead to:

1. Reliance on praise to feel good enough
2. A need to feel superior to others to feel good enough
3. Inflated self-importance
4. Unrealistic expectations of praise outside the home
5. An unrealistic sense of entitlement in the real world
6. Feelings of disappointment and failure when praise is not received
7. Preoccupation with earning praise rather than pursuing authentic interests
8. Avoiding important pursuits, such as healthy experimentation and hard work, that do not win immediate praise
9. Attributing success to innate ability rather than effort
10. Expecting immediate rather than earned rewards
11. Valuing rewards over experience itself
12. Valuing outcomes over learning
13. Valuing innate talent over hard work and practice
14. Valuing praise and entitlement over internal satisfaction
15. Fear and avoidance of appearing ordinary
16. Feelings of threat, shame, and rage at neutral or critical responses

17. Overreliance on others' assessments for self-esteem
18. A dysregulated sense of reality
19. The belief that only praiseworthy outcomes lead to acceptance and love
20. Equating success with worthiness and praise with love

Looking at this list, we see that excessively praised children, especially ones who are also directly or indirectly devalued for certain other qualities, take on narcissistic patterns of feeling and thinking about themselves and others. They become addicted to exaggerated self-beliefs and react with shame and rage when those beliefs are threatened. Anything less than constant praise may come to feel like failure and attack. Overpraised children become isolated from and at odds with their peers because in the culture of their families they must be better than them to be good enough. They measure their self-worth based on what wins praise and avoid exploring or expressing parts of themselves that don't, narrowing the shape of their life to parameters set externally by others.

THE PAIN OF THE PARENTIFIED CHILD

When Adam was growing up, his narcissistic mother insisted on perfection from him, her eldest child. By fourth grade, he was expected to get straight A's. Anything less unleashed violent rage, hysteria that he wouldn't get into college, and assigned readings of an encyclopedia.

As Adam got older, Fridays after school were chore nights until ten p.m. His father was usually at night school, and his mother would call from work to dictate a list of jobs. Adam learned to roast a chicken, clean the house, pay the bills, and take care of his little brother. Soon his mother was dropping him off to do the grocery shopping. "At 12, I thought it was really cool that I could do that," he said.

Like so many parentified children, for Adam being given adult responsibilities and learning to handle them well was a source of pride. Now he looks back with hurt and anger: "I have felt like the adult in this family for as long as I can remember." Yet, as is common among hero kids, he remains confused now, at 38, about whether he asked for the responsibilities or was unfairly burdened with them, despite his therapist's assurances that his circumstances were abusive and not within his control.

Also typical of children of narcissistic parents, Adam became hypervigilant: "I used to sit in the house and listen when my mother got home for how the car door slammed, the tone of her walk on the pavement, to gauge her mood." He also learned to hide his needs, such as the time he was pretending to be a knight. "I had put a fillet knife in a sheath, and when I pulled it out, I sliced my hand to the bone. Blood was everywhere." Fearing his mother's anger, he wrapped his hand in thick cotton and stayed in his room.

When Adam's mother wasn't venting anger and blame, she resorted to silent treatment and stonewalling. "If I disagreed or did anything that was remotely like a child, she would go silent for days. She wouldn't respond or make meals," he said. "To this day I get really flustered if people are unresponsive. I turn red and get intensely anxious."

By age 13, as Adam was realizing he was gay, his father moved out temporarily and his mother responded by retreating to her room. "She just shut down and cried all the time," he said. "I understand now that I had to step up caretaking my mother and brother at a time when I needed support for coming out." Adam struggles with his father's enabling role in the family. "I'm learning to be pissed at my dad. He doesn't have a mean bone in his body. But I'm learning that when you are a human who mates with another human there is 50-50 responsibility. My mother dominated, and my father didn't push back. He still tells me not to burden her if anything is going on with me."

Despite professional success and years of personal work, including therapy, yoga, and retreats, Adam is still plagued with panic attacks, chronic digestive problems, addiction, anger, and difficulty with trust. He said, "I haven't had an intimate relationship for five years. I'm digging all this stuff up, identifying the emotional abuse. It's hard to reach out."

Regarding his relationship with his parents now, Adam is working to assert boundaries but feels ambivalent. "My therapist says I need to stop talking to them. But Mom has a brain disease and my brother is dealing with serious problems. My character is to not check out on my family. You're biologically dictated to crawl back to reconcile," he said.

Adam has struggled for years to acknowledge his family experience as abuse since he wasn't physically harmed. His is a common confusion for emotionally and psychologically abused children, especially parentified ones who identify as strong and capable. "There is something specifically insidious about the non-physical abuse," he said. "It's such a weird pathology, one of the hardest things to treat. I'm in the midst of heavy depression, while my close friends look to me to be functional and caretaking. The truth is I want to latch onto someone to save me, but I know it doesn't work that way. All we want is to be loved." «

THE TRAP OF THE EMOTIONAL CARETAKER

Meredith grew up with a depressed narcissistic mother and an intermittently absent and overbearing narcissistic father. Her mother was at times loving and fun but suffered from insecurity and depression. Her mother's father had been cruel to her and favored her brother, and her mother had been passive and distant. "When my mother married my father, she continued the cycle. He constantly criticized and gaslighted her," Meredith explained.

Meredith became her mother's support system, the person she turned to for companionship and reassurance. "Her extreme neediness came out in the form of jealousy whenever I would go out with my friends or try to have a life of my own," she said. "She would act offended and hurt, and I would feel guilty." Meredith recalled a terrifying incident when she was little: "My mother locked herself in the bathroom and said she was going to kill herself because no one loved her and we'd be better off without her. I was afraid from that moment on that she would do that, and it was my responsibility to keep her alive."

Over the years Meredith's mother continued to threaten suicide and her father would huff in disgust and leave home for months. "It was too complicated for me to manage having relationships other than with her. My only friends were people I would hang out with at school when she couldn't expect me to be at home. When I was little, my father and I whistled together and played sometimes, but my mother made it clear I had to make a choice between them, and that choice had to be her," Meredith explained. She said her childhood felt like a jail sentence, and during high school she was counting down the days until she could leave home.

As a young adult, Meredith sought therapy and was fortunate to find someone who identified her parents' narcissism. "I worked hard for the next four years to understand their issues. I had a long way to go, but that was the beginning of my recovery," she said. When her mother (by then separated from her father) followed her to the city where she had relocated, Meredith was in her late 20s and had gained enough perspective to draw boundaries so that they could have a workable relationship.

"I was able to assert my independence and come back to my mother with compassion. I knew she wasn't out to hurt me—that was never her goal. Since I had my son she has been involved in our lives in positive ways, but if there is something wrong like I'm having an [rheumatoid] arthritis flare-up or she's upset with my father, I have to talk her off the ledge." «

seventeen

Understanding and Overcoming Your Family Role

NARCISSISTIC PARENTS ASSIGN ROLES TO THEIR CHILDREN TO CONTROL family dynamics and reinforce their deluded self-beliefs. Like other aspects of the narcissistic family, child roles are artificial and meant to serve the needs of the parents rather than support the children's authenticity and development. The parents interpret reality not as it is but as they need and wish it to be, and the kids are expected to play along without question or suffer the consequences. Children defined by artificial roles experience distortions to their sense of identity and face emotional and psychological trauma that can last a lifetime if not addressed.

THE USUAL SUSPECTS: CHILD ROLES AND HOW THEY ARE ASSIGNED

As in other types of dysfunctional families, children in the narcissistic family fall into the common roles of scapegoat, lost child, mascot, and variations of hero that may blend with the scapegoat role. But narcissistic families differ in that there is nearly always an idealized golden child, a role that also may blend with aspects of the hero. I discuss these child roles in Chapters 8 and 15; here, I examine their implications for adult children of narcissists.

Narcissistic parents assign the different roles to particular children for a range of reasons, both calculating and unconscious and always self-serving. Oftentimes, children are given roles based on birth order, gender, or whether they remind a narcissistic parent of her-/himself in "bad" or "good" ways. The roles of scapegoat and golden child are primary roles in the family that are usually given to first and second children. In larger families, a third child may take on the mascot mantle, but later assume the lost child role if a fourth child is born and becomes the mascot. Roles also may shift when children leave home or when there are other changes such as divorce. Children with two families sometimes play different roles in each home. Children in single-child families may fall in and out of different roles for periods of time or even day to day.

SCAPEGOAT

Narcissists always need a target, and the scapegoated child is it. Blamed for the ills of the family, scapegoats are treated to negative projection, criticism, and rage and are often burdened with excessive responsibilities as well as restrictions at home. If you are a scapegoat, no matter how hard you try or how capable you are, it is seldom good enough, and anything negative you do is viewed as proof of your failings. You are labeled a screw-up or rebel so that any reaction you have against the injustice of the role can always be interpreted as confirmation of its accuracy. As the family bad seed, whether you try to explain, argue, yell, cry, or withdraw, it is seen as acting out. In a very real sense, as scapegoat you experience a character assassination that may amount to a lifelong smear campaign within the family and possibly beyond it to relatives, friends, and community members.

The child selected for scapegoating triggers the parent's narcissistic injury, activating her/his most violent defenses. Your mere act of seeing causes the parent to lash out with projecting rage: You are called difficult, unfair, angry, disloyal. The narcissist's disappointments become your fault. The narcissist's abuses become your misdeeds. The narcissist's responsibilities become your weights to carry. In short, the narcissistic parent uses you to deflect accountability and as a catchall for her/his disappointments and anger at the world.

As the family target, you as scapegoat have it hardest, at least on the surface. Your narcissistic parent sees in you what s/he hates about her-/himself. This may be because you are most like that parent, most aware of her/his shortcomings, and/or most questioning of or confrontational about the family's unhealthy dynamics. Perhaps you are the most aware and/or strongest child and therefore the biggest threat to the narcissist's architecture of lies.

Scapegoated children may react at home and school by fulfilling their role as underachiever, disaffected misfit, or rule-breaking rebel. They may struggle against family expectations by taking on aspects of the hero role, becoming hyperresponsible and perfectionist overachievers and/or self-effacing caregivers/rescuers. They may internalize the narcissistic value system and become narcissistic themselves, reacting to feelings of shame with grandiose and controlling compensations. Sometimes scapegoated children endure so much assault that they experience a kind of emotional and/or physical collapse that leaves them unable to fully function in adulthood. In extreme cases, scapegoats are so pathologized they end up institutionalized or homeless. However they respond to their circumstances, scapegoats inevitably carry the emotional and physical fallout of abuse. As long-term trauma victims, they are most likely to experience symptoms of CPTSD, including anxiety, depression, anger, phobias, addiction, and degraded health. Those who avoid becoming narcissistic themselves are vulnerable to codependent and/or abusive relationships, especially if an enabling parent has modeled codependency.

But scapegoats' vulnerabilities are often also their most powerful strengths. As a scapegoat, you may become highly empathetic, having been marginalized and trained to put others' needs first. You also may become unusually self-reflective, seeking out insight and awareness to make sense of the abuse and cognitive dissonance you endured. As an outlier, you are likely to have greater perspective about the family dysfunction and motivation to break away from it. If you are able to carry such awareness forward into healthier relationships, you may end the cycle of blame and abuse with your own family. Often it takes having kids of our own to realize how far out of bounds our parents were with us. Scapegoats who become parents commonly experience an aha moment (or many moments) when they say, "I would *never* treat my kids the way my parents treated me!"[1]

Like the golden child, as scapegoat your identity is distorted by the narcissistic parent's false projections. Your challenge is to believe in your own perceptions and truths—no small matter for someone who has been undermined in a devastating smear campaign. This means dissecting the narcissistic family system, recognizing its cruelties and lies, and nurturing the self within who was never properly loved.

GOLDEN CHILD

The golden child is the privileged family favorite whose strengths and successes are celebrated and failings are typically overlooked or blamed on the scapegoat. This child serves as a projection of what the dominant narcissistic parent wants to believe about her-/himself. As the object of idealized attention, the golden child's identity becomes deeply enmeshed with the parent's at the expense of the child's own normal individuation and personal development. Such a child becomes closely attuned to that parent's emotions, learning to conform to that parent's needs while burying her/his own.

The golden child may take on a caregiver role with the parent, building her/his identity around pleasing. Or such a child may work to perform well in areas valued by the parents, such as athletics or academics. Like children in the hero role, golden children often feel pressure to excel and present well for the family, working hard to distinguish themselves and becoming perfectionist to maintain their entitled status.

Although the golden child is usually shielded from the narcissist's worst offenses and elevated in the family hierarchy, that privilege comes at a cost. The narcissistic parent charges a high price for her/his favoritism: isolation and compliance. If you are that parent's golden child, s/he "owns" you and demands your attention, adulation, and loyalty. As a result, you may feel overresponsible for that parent as well as smothered, controlled, and isolated. Other family members may resent or withdraw from you, and you may feel guilty about your entitlement or become perfectionist and overachieving to maintain it. You may become arrogant and intolerant but also insecure about who you feel you really are, adopting your parent's narcissism. If you attempt to break away from the narcissist's dominance or form independent relationships, you will likely face reprisal, from guilt trips to judgment, threats to ostracism.

It can be harder to see the damage done to those cast in the golden child role than those scapegoated. They appear to be above reproach—adored, excused, and often coddled. But, like scapegoats, golden children are merely pawns in the narcissistic family system, extensions of the narcissist with undeveloped identities and few personal boundaries of their own. What appears to be favoritism is a form of emotional imprisonment.

Often golden children are pushed to examine their family dynamics when they get married or have kids of their own. Their parents may scapegoat their partner or children or scapegoat them instead of a formerly scapegoated sibling. This may shift the golden child's view of things and force her/him to face the family dysfunction. What was hidden by denial and privileged status may feel shockingly revealed and trigger a reassessment of the past and a reordering of the present. At such a juncture, adult golden children may decide to limit contact or withdraw altogether to protect themselves or their current families.

As an adult golden child, life's realities are likely to run interference with your confusing mix of overconfidence and underlying self-doubt. You may experience cognitive dissonance at having outsiders treat you as ordinary after your family has treated you as extraordinary. You may struggle with under- or overachievement, too afraid of failing to fully try or too perfectionist to ever feel successful enough. You are likely to feel angry about the burdens placed on you by your selfish and demanding parent, but still struggle with the compulsion to conform and appease those in positions of authority. Your ability to have healthy independent relationships requires a willingness to establish boundaries with your parents and move beyond your prescribed role, including giving up its entitlements. Your most difficult challenges are overcoming a sense of instilled helplessness, setting realistic expectations for yourself, and gaining an appropriate sense of self-importance in the scheme of things. More than anything, you need to feel validated and loved for who you are rather than what you represent to your parent or anyone else.

LOST CHILD

Often a third child, the lost child is effectively overshadowed by the golden child, while spared the brunt of the wrath directed at the scapegoat. By the time this child appears, the family is distracted by the drama around the other two roles and has little use for a newcomer. Often, lost children carry around the belief that they are family afterthoughts, with no rightful claim. Unwilling or unable to compete, lost children withdraw from the chaos both emotion-ally and physically. They often spend time alone doing solitary activities. Even when with other family members, they become masters at disappearing in plain sight. For lost children, no attention is better than any kind of atten-tion. This applies at school as well as at home, where they tend to moderate everything they do and blend in like well-camouflaged animals of prey.

As the lost child, avoidance and dissociation are your main defenses. While this helps you disengage from negative drama and evade being targeted, it also means sacrificing self-awareness, emotional growth, and intimacy with others.

Having learned to self-efface, as an adult you don't know how to be the protagonist in your own story. You are so accustomed to receding into the background that calling attention to yourself in any way makes you feel dangerously exposed. You have interests and talents, but it has always felt unsafe to take them seriously. You may find yourself unsure of what you want and reluctant to fully commit to a career or relationship. You may long for closeness with others but don't know how to reach out and fear being seen as needy, selfish, or demanding. Because you find it difficult to connect, you may feel lonely or overly dependent on a few trusted people.

To heal past wounds, it is important to focus on your feelings and build self-awareness. Practice identifying your needs and preferences and express-ing them in your relationships. Take risks you would have avoided before, such as reaching out socially or pursuing an interest. Getting to know your-self, developing your talents and passions, and making personal connections are important building blocks for self-confidence and well-being.

MASCOT

The mascot is the child who provides entertaining distraction and comic relief from the family dysfunction. Typically the youngest child, the mascot is the court jester who hams it up to get attention and diffuse tension. This child may be spoiled and given relatively free license at home, while being allowed to coast or get in trouble at school. Often class clowns and come-dians, mascots can be well liked and popular or in some cases overly kinetic and demanding to be around. They tend to avoid leadership roles and take longer than others to mature.

Because mascots are young, not taken seriously, and not privy to things other older family members know, they are often plagued with feelings of confusion, anxiety, and helplessness. Relying on their ability to entertain, mascots can become compulsively attention seeking while not knowing how to think for themselves and handle age-appropriate responsibilities. Like lost children, mascots typically have a deficit of self-awareness. Socially, they may have surface confidence, but this masks deeper insecurities, anger, and the tendency to deny and dissociate from emotions.

As a mascot, you probably have difficulty listening to your feelings and trusting your abilities. Because you are externally focused, you may struggle to be organized, stay on task, and be fully in your body. You are vulnerable to escapist and avoidant distractions, including addictive behavior. In relationships, you may feel responsible for other people's happiness in ways that are overwhelming for you, and your habit of sublimating your needs can lead to codependency. Making others laugh can be rewarding, but as a compulsive mask for pain it can create feelings of emptiness, isolation, and despair.

As a mascot child in adulthood, one of your core issues is overcoming your impulse to deny and redirect uncomfortable or painful emotions. Connecting with your feelings and honoring them with the respect they deserve is important to gain inner equilibrium. Look for ways to ground yourself through physical activity and self-reflection. Tap into your natural empathy, and build trust and intimacy in your relationships through direct and honest communication. Challenge yourself to take on leadership roles at home and work to reinforce your sense of competency. Learning to slow down, be present with yourself, take your needs seriously, and believe in your abilities are roads to healing.

A MASTER MANAGER MASCOT

The youngest of four siblings/stepsiblings in both her mother's and father's homes, Brook played the cute, funny charmer who found a way to relate to everyone and get her needs met outside her family at the houses of friends. Because she placed few demands on her parents, often lying to appease them, they came to view her as their "easy" and "well-adjusted" child. As she got older, Brook was drawn to high-drama friends and partners and prided herself on being able to manage all kinds of personalities, especially difficult ones. But she also struggled with feeling overextended socially and drained by her relationships, often feigning illness so she could be alone and recover.

As some of her siblings worked on understanding the family dysfunction and setting boundaries with their parents, Brook believed she had been so skilled at managing her family that she had avoided the trauma her siblings were struggling with. "I was concerned that I had big blank spots in my memory of my childhood, but I believed I was in control and could handle things my siblings just couldn't," she said. Brook started to see things differently when she and her husband began fighting bitterly about his parents. "My in-laws adored me, and my husband was the identified patient who they said was lucky to have me. Our marriage counselor helped me see that his parents were scapegoating him and I was playing into it."

As Brook explored her past in therapy she realized that believing she had managed her parents and escaped their abuse was a form of denial. "I had to accept that I was not immune from harm and that my success at handling people was actually keeping me from being honest with myself and facing my own vulnerability," she explained. "Now I'm getting closer to my husband and remembering more of my childhood, which is hard but not as scary as having it buried," she explained. "I'm drinking less and learning to be present and not dissociate when I'm stressed." <<

A GOLDEN CHILD'S ISOLATION AND GUILT

Janine grew up with a verbally assaultive narcissist father. Her mother and two older brothers were scapegoated, while she was her father's treasured favorite. As an adult in her 50s, she came across a description of the narcissist's "golden child." She said, "When I read it I just froze. It was me."

As early as Janine could remember, her father went on rage binges, spending hours and even days at a time stomping around the house, berating her mother and brothers. "Something so innocuous would trigger it. He would find a reason to go off," Janine said. "It was so loud you could hear it on the road. I know the neighbors could hear it. He would go on for hours and hours, yelling, ranting, 'You did this, you did that.' I had such shame about it. At the time, it was overwhelming."

As his favorite, Janine went hiking with her father and shared long talks. She thought if she could make the day good, everything would be okay when they got home. She was never at ease, never sure when the next explosion would come. "I had to be happy and cheerful all the time. You're playing a role. You're not really you."

Inevitably, her father's temper flared at the rest of her family. Sometimes, he threw her brothers out of the house. "They'd be out in the rain in their socks," Janine remembered. "My mother would sit in a chair, huddled over, sometimes pretending to read. She figured out not to fight because it would make things worse. Sometimes she would take us away. Once we stayed in a hotel."

Janine said about her mother and brothers, "It didn't make any sense; they were wonderful humans. My brothers are talented musicians, much more talented than I am. I had very strong feelings of guilt. I watched the people I loved receive the rage. I felt like I should have been able to fix things. My mother would tell me to go to my room and be very, very quiet."

Although Janine was spared her father's direct wrath, she was around during the worst years of his abuse. "Being the youngest, I think I might have been more affected," she said. "My brothers are six and eight years older. I think they had happier earlier years because the marriage was better then, and they had each other and left home as soon as they could. I had all those years alone wanting to fix it, seeing my father's abuse of my mother."

Janine described her mother as loving and adventurous and a talented painter. She turned to Christian Science for meaning in her life, but in time suffered from an untreated case of pneumonia that eventually killed her in her 60s. A man Janine was involved with at the time said it was her mother's way of committing suicide. "It was shocking to hear him say that, but the essence of it was true," Janine said. "We were devastated when she died."

Typical of golden children, Janine grew up feeling isolated, both from her family members and socially. She worried that her mother resented her. "I felt, 'My god, why can't you be nice to Mom like you are to me?' You become over-sensitized to those around you because your life depends on it." Her middle brother told her jokingly, "Yeah, we just ignored you." Janine stopped having friends over after one asked to go home because her father was yelling.

Also typical of golden children, Janine felt disturbingly engulfed by her father. She said there were no clear boundaries between them. "Sometimes he would refer to me as his 'girlfriend.' I didn't like it. He felt too much for me in a way that a dad shouldn't. It's not like a father's love should feel. It felt wrong, like emotional incest."

Janine left home early and married a verbally and physically abusive narcissist whom she had dated since she was 14, flip-flopping her role as golden child to brutalized scapegoat. She said, "He tore me down so much he literally had me on my knees."

She was plagued with low self-esteem and health problems starting in her 20s, including a diagnosis of multiple sclerosis. When Janine told her father about her MS, he replied, "People with MS like to blame other people for all their problems." After leaving her first marriage, she endured a second abusive relationship. Through years of therapy, she eventually made her way into a loving marriage.

Janine said one of her most healing experiences happened in therapy when she was confronted with her feelings about herself as a child. "I realized I had extreme hatred for that little girl. The beginning of my healing was becoming compassionate to that little person who had no power. The beginning of the journey was forgiving myself for not being able to save my family." <<

eighteen

Sibling Relationships

SIBLING RELATIONSHIPS ARE COMPLICATED EVEN IN THE HAPPIEST OF homes, and a certain degree of sibling rivalry is normal. Sibling experiences within families can vary significantly, depending on personality differences, gender, birth order, and other circumstances, such as finances, relocation, illness, and divorce. In the turbulent narcissistic home, family members are constantly under siege and struggling to cope. In some cases, especially where there is significant neglect, siblings may band together and in essence raise each other, forging supportive bonds to survive. But more typically, siblings in such conditions become competitive and alienated, if not combative, because of

- limited emotional and perhaps physical resources,
- the constant selfish demands of the narcissistic parent(s),
- the constant threat of emotional and/or physical harm, and
- divisions deliberately created by the parent(s).

WHY NARCISSISTIC PARENTS DIVIDE THEIR CHILDREN

Unlike stable, loving parents who strive to create a cohesive and nurturing family environment for everyone, narcissistic parents disrupt and undermine relationships among family members. That includes relationships among children and other nonnarcissistic parents/stepparents, relationships between immediate and extended family, and relationships among siblings.

Sowing division may be a deliberate means of control, or it may be collateral damage in NPD parents' pursuit of getting their needs met regardless of the consequences for others. The bottom line is that narcissists do not care whether their kids love and respect one another and often see more benefit to themselves in ensuring that the children don't.

1. They Feel Threatened

At the most basic level, narcissists are threatened by other people's relationships, particularly those among their kids. This is because they

- view life as a zero-sum game in which they can only "win" by causing someone else to lose;
- want attention and resources for themselves and view sharing as deprivation;
- are incapable of the give-and-take of authentic intimacy and don't want others to have something they don't have;
- fear losing control over their kids' thoughts, feelings, and actions; and
- most important, fear the power of a unified front.

2. They Are Binary Thinkers

As we have discussed, narcissists view themselves and others in simplistic, either/or terms, as all good or all bad, right or wrong, successful or a failure, with little territory in between. When it comes to their kids, they typically idealize and favor one and reject and devalue another. One is talented and the other is a disappointment, one is brilliant and the other is average or stupid, one is above reproach and the other is to blame when things go wrong. Although there is typically an ongoing pattern of idealizing a particular child and devaluing another, narcissistic parents usually also experience short-term vacillations from hour to hour or day to day in how they see their kids, with the pendulum swinging from one child to another so that favoritism shifts. This may happen if narcissists feel disappointed in their golden child or impressed with something the scapegoat, lost child, or mascot has done, leading them to devalue a generally elevated daughter or son because they cannot hold both children in the same "good" category in their mind and must relegate one to the "bad" category.

3. They Want Control

Narcissists seek to control others to gain attention and uphold their mask of exceptionalism and entitlement. Their children must be brought to heel in sustaining their grandiose pretense with whatever means necessary. Weakening sibling bonds and pitting children against one another is a virtual inevitability in the narcissistic home.

THE DIVIDE-AND-CONQUER STRATEGY

As in any totalitarian regime, the dictatorial narcissistic parent attempts to exact compliance from her/his children both physically and psychologically, controlling not just their behavior but also their thoughts. Sibling alliances threaten narcissists' control and are undermined in a divide-and-conquer strategy of breaking down power into isolated, more manageable pieces. Narcissistic parents engineer rivalries and pit siblings against one another through inequitable conditions, ranking and comparing, negative propaganda, playing favorites, and triangulation.

1. Inequitable Conditions

By setting up disparities in how they treat their children, parents in a narcissistic home create a power imbalance among siblings that breeds resentment. They may grant privileges, such as freedom, money, or exemption from chores, to one child and not another. One child may be allowed to go out or choose her/his own clothing while another child is restricted. One child may be given spending money or gifts, while another gets less or nothing. One child may be assigned few to no duties around the house, while another is burdened with excessive responsibilities. Such inequities establish a power hierarchy in the narcissistic family that leaves some children higher in the pecking order than others and fosters conflict.

2. Ranking and Comparing

By ranking and comparing their kids, narcissistic parents create a competitive environment at home that keeps siblings vying with one another for praise and a reprieve from judgment and ridicule. One child is always up, while another is down. One is tougher, prettier, or more popular, while another is weak, unattractive, or friendless. As long as kids are competing, the parents wield control.

3. Negative Propaganda

Any totalitarian state uses propaganda as a means of mind control, and the narcissistic home is no different. To sow divisions among siblings, narcissistic parents *sell ideas* about their kids, ideas that are distorted and often have no basis in reality. A child who questions such parents may be labeled angry and rebellious, while one who accepts their narrative is loyal and trustworthy. Narcissistic parents use propaganda to label their kids and influence how the kids perceive themselves and one another. Because such messages are established very early in children's lives, they are especially pernicious and difficult to break free from.

4. Playing Favorites

Along with setting up inequitable conditions and ranking and comparing, narcissistic parents create jealousy and infighting among their kids by playing favorites. One child is granted attention and praise, while another is ignored or shamed. One is idealized as the can-do-no-wrong golden child, and another is devalued as the can-do-no-right scapegoat. By holding one child in favor and another in disfavor, such parents create a polarity between siblings that positions them in opposition to each other and places themselves in the power role of judge. Even scapegoats may be favored at times in the daily ebb and flow of life in the narcissistic home, keeping them and other children off balance and in the game.

Common Idealizing Behaviors
1. Flattery
2. Excessive attention
3. Gifts
4. Exaggerated praise
5. Bragging to others
6. Mirroring
7. Seduction/sexualization

8. "Positive" projection
9. Exemption from responsibility and/or accountability
10. Special privileges

Common Devaluing Behaviors

1. Criticism
2. Blame
3. Mockery and ridicule, often presented as "teasing"
4. Negative projection
5. Lies and denial
6. Neglect
7. Terror
8. Gaslighting
9. Excessive responsibilities
10. Smear campaigns

5. Triangulation

Narcissistic parents triangulate family interactions as a means of controlling the flow and content of communication between their kids. In this three-party dynamic, narcissists' goal is to act as the primary channel of conversation while keeping the kids isolated from one another. This way, they can manipulate what and how much is said, to keep the focus of importance upon themselves and drive a wedge between siblings. Narcissistic puppet masters thrive on triangulation and regard direct communication between siblings as a threat.

COPING WITH THE GOLDEN CHILD SIBLING

For children in the narcissistic family, dealing with a golden child sibling is often frustrating and painful. They may love their favored brother or sister and seek her/his attention and approval, only to be met with judgment and betrayal. Siblings, especially the scapegoat, may experience tattling or bullying from a golden child without understanding why. They may feel angry and resentful about the family inequity and withdraw to protect themselves. Particularly if the golden child adopts the narcissistic parent's attitudes and behavior, there may be little to nothing that siblings can do to create trust or closeness with that brother or sister. As we have just discussed, parents are often well aware of such dynamics and play into their children's insecurities, magnifying alienation among their kids. Children under such circumstances at best disengage from and at worst prey on one another, with the golden child typically in the abuser role.

SIBLING RELATIONSHIPS IN ADULTHOOD

Sibling relationships in a narcissistic family nearly inevitably suffer the fallout of the destructive scenarios orchestrated by their emotionally disturbed parents. Even where there is affection and concern, there is often also alienation and possibly outright conflict that is typically perpetuated into adulthood. In many families, adult children persist in believing the distortions they grew up with and continue to play out patterns of distrust, discord, and perhaps betrayal. This is more likely to be the case if the parents are still dominating the family and influencing sibling interactions through triangulation and competition over resources, such as money. Adult children who recognize the dysfunction and work to overcome parental control may succeed in forming alliances and developing independent connections among their own families.

Dissecting the narcissistic parents' sick and self-serving messages, understanding the suffering of sisters and brothers in the narcissistic family system, and communicating directly can help repair the damage and provide desperately needed validation. But efforts to connect with adult siblings should be made with caution, since many children adopt their disordered parents' narcissistic patterns of thought and behavior and may be untrustworthy and beyond reach later in life. For adult children who have gained insight into narcissistic family dynamics, accepting that their siblings are unreachable can be one of the most painful things to come to terms with. Adult siblings abused by a golden child have good reason to pull away and limit or end contact. But for siblings who can overcome denial and constricting family roles, renewed closeness in adulthood can be powerfully validating. For everyone involved, compassion balanced with self-advocacy is the road to acceptance and healing.

LOST AND FOUND SISTERS

Lottie and her sister, Pippin, had been close as little kids, but grew apart because of tensions between them related to the roles they played in their family. Lottie was often scapegoated, while Pippin disappeared into the lost child role. Their half brother Mick was their father's golden child, who bullied his sisters and was not disciplined. As adults, the sisters began to talk about their childhood. When Lottie told Pippin she was hurt that Pippin pulled away from her, Pippin was able to explain things from her perspective. "I reminded Lottie that when I had tried to defend her with our brother it just made Dad angrier at her. And Mick would torment both of us when we spent time together because he was jealous of our relationship. It felt safer to just keep to myself," Pippin said. Both sisters talked about how painful things had been, and Lottie was able to get support for how she had been scapegoated. Lottie said, "We finally shared what things were like for us. It was incredible to know that Pippin understood what I went through and to understand her experience better." «

CHARLOTTE'S WEB

Charlotte was 7 when she became in her words the "death dealer" on her family's makeshift farm. At her mother's insistence, the family moved from the city and embarked on a grand experiment as do-it-yourself farmers.

Charlotte's first time watching chicks hatch lurched from delighted wonder to a harsh lesson in the dirty work of farming and a prescribed part in the family script that would shape her life. After one of the chicks emerged deformed and quivering with its stomach outside of its skin, Charlotte's mother leaned into her daughter, just home from second grade, and hissed, "Get rid of it—it won't live." When Charlotte asked what she should do with the misshapen chick, her mother snapped, "Figure it out!"

Charlotte was good at figuring things out, and her resourcefulness made her the go-to "superkid" in a family with two narcissistic parents: an abusive mother who hit, insulted, rejected, and neglected her two daughters and an absent, self-centered father who used passive-aggressive manipulation to get his way.

Charlotte said her older sister, Maggie, adopted "learned helplessness" to cope, while Charlotte became hyperresponsible. "Our mother smacked me around more, but she criticized Maggie more, constantly telling her she was useless. Maggie went 'spaghetti legs,' so I was the one who had to deal with stuff."

Charlotte's appointed role as hero/scapegoat became a terrifying matter of survival when she came upon her mother slaughtering a pig one day. "She had suspended a large boar upside down in a tree," Charlotte said. "Blood was filling a bucket below a gaping slash in his throat. Entrails were spilling out like snakes. The other pigs were screaming. She yanked on my arm and told me, 'Shut up and do what I tell you, or you go in that tree with it.'"

Faced with botched castrations, fumbled births, interrupted fox attacks, and "butcheries gone horribly wrong," Charlotte became the family finisher, the one who completed the job, no matter how gruesome, and buried the dead. "I was accurate with a pistol and hatchet, strong for my age. I had to be. It takes a lot of digging to bury a 2,000-pound cow. As I looked into her huge liquid eyes, I felt guilt and shame at what I was made to do—and terror over what would happen to me if I didn't," she said.

Charlotte's father was gone a lot, working a job with a long commute. At home, Charlotte said, he fought constantly with her mother, who vented her anger at her kids and slipped into alcoholism. "Dad was clingy with my mother, but also critical of her—he was a dependent narcissist who wanted attention and needed everyone to do things for him," she said.

Charlotte said her father turned a blind eye to his wife's abuse of the kids and didn't have time for her unless he needed to vent about her mother. "I remember once he took me for a drive and started crying about Mom. I was terrified, because I was maybe 6 or 7 and had no idea what he was talking about. He was so out of control. I needed him to be the adult, and he was looking to a child for comfort. Thinking back on it makes me want to vomit. He didn't touch me, but it felt like emotional incest."

Charlotte's father continued to parentify her until at about 16 she told him she would no longer listen to him talk about her mother. Around the same time, when she was finally the same height as her mother, she stood up to her mother's raised hand and said, "Are you really gonna hit me?"

Charlotte's mother's abuse lessened somewhat after that, but her father continued to bait and manipulate Charlotte. "He told rude jokes and tried to convince me to convert to this extremely bigoted church he'd joined." Now, decades later and several years since Charlotte severely limited contact with her father, he still sends her racist and sexist spam, she said, "to elicit a response."

When Charlotte was 11, her brother was born. Her father announced, "A son! I finally got it right." By then Charlotte was doing most of the cooking and laundry, paying bills, and fielding calls from creditors. She started caring for her brother when her mother complained that he was "a screamy baby."

Charlotte said, "My plan was to graduate early and go in the military for school and freedom. But I put my plan aside to look after my brother because I was afraid of what could happen to him."

Her little brother quickly became the family golden child, indulged and absolved from responsibility. Their father in particular infantilized him, over-looking it when his son would steal from the family, not making him do chores, giving him cars and bailing him out of jail.

"I resented my brother, but what made me most angry was how my father made him helpless," Charlotte said. "My father needed to be needed. He never encouraged his son to go to college. Dad has him and his girlfriend and their kids set up in a house next to his. My brother doesn't know how to hold down a job. His girlfriend has never worked. Dad made him arrogant, but he didn't give him confidence."

Charlotte eventually left home and worked her way through college and then graduate school, the first in her family to do so. In time, she went into the field of counseling. "I didn't consciously pursue it as a way to heal myself, but I've found that the most valuable part of my work has been the unex-pected benefit of gaining education and insight about my family dynamics and spreading this to others. This insight has allowed me to see that I did not cause these events and that as a child I was an innocent in this chaos, simply trying to survive."

Like so many children of narcissists, Charlotte and her sister have struggled with self-esteem and health problems that Charlotte believes are related to early trauma. Charlotte has had symptoms of CPTSD, an autoimmune thyroid disease, polycystic ovary syndrome, fibromyalgia, and gallstones. Neither sister had children for fear of continuing the family legacy.

Charlotte counts herself fortunate too, especially knowing she is helping people from similar circumstances in her practice: "Having the ability to sup-port and validate the experiences of others as they break free is a gift. While I realize there is no karmic balance sheet, I feel a purpose when I can help 'even the score' bit by bit, person by person, as they pull themselves up and out." ‹‹

PART 6

OVERCOMING NARCISSISTIC ABUSE

nineteen

Processing Your Trauma

A S SOMEONE WHO HAS ENDURED NARCISSISTIC ABUSE, YOU FIND
yourself feeling broken and grappling with painful questions. Why
did it take so long to identify the damage? Why didn't others help more?
How could the brutalizing cycle play and replay so many times? Perhaps
you are 30, 40, 50, 60, or older, having carried the weight of grief for many
years.

WHY OVERCOMING NARCISSISTIC
ABUSE TRAUMA TAKES SO LONG

Contrary to what we are often taught to believe, there is no strict life
schedule for any of us. We all learn and grow at different rates in different areas of our lives. Understanding an abusive relationship, particularly
one with a narcissist, is especially difficult because of the complex trauma
surrounding it. For most of us, healing from trauma is a long slow slog:
three steps forward, one step back, and one step sideways. It is common
for childhood trauma sufferers to remain in a survivalist state of denial and
self-blame well into middle adulthood or longer.[1] Until recently, there was
limited public understanding of narcissism and narcissistic abuse trauma
and even less information about how to manage it. Moreover, people's understanding of trauma and treating it, particularly long-term trauma, is still
in many ways in its infancy.

Here are other reasons recovering from narcissistic abuse is such a slow process.

1. Narcissistic Abuse Is Hidden

Narcissists often go to great lengths to conceal their abusive behavior and project an ideal image of themselves and their life to the outside world. They are, in essence, all about projection—image rather than substance, and they guilt, shame, and bully those around them into supporting their sham reality. Their family members are continuously pressured to comply with their demands and uphold the distorted version of the family that the narcissists insist on, regardless of the harm it does to all involved. Often, they gaslight and browbeat their partner into enabling their behavior, making the harm to the family that much harder to call out.

2. Narcissistic Abuse Is Hard to Believe

In addition to being hidden from public view, narcissistic abuse is so far beyond the bounds of normal behavior that it is hard to believe, even for those subjected to it. People without direct experience with narcissism have little to no reference point for understanding narcissists' grotesquely inflated self-importance, outsize need for attention and admiration, and pathological lack of empathy. One need look no further than the catastrophic abuses of such malignant narcissist tyrants as Joseph Stalin, Adolf Hitler, Saddam Hussein,[2] Pol Pot, and Idi Amin[3] to understand just how far narcissists can go and how much they are allowed to get away with.

3. Narcissistic Abuse Trains You to Blame Yourself

A hallmark of narcissism is refusing accountability and blaming others, particularly victims. By blaming a targeted victim for their abusive behavior, narcissists deflect responsibility and further weaken the target's defenses. The best-case scenario for narcissists is to be able to manipulate and abuse freely without consequence, and conditioning victims to blame themselves is the most effective way to ensure their compliance. For children in the narcissistic family, unlearning the habit of self-blame is particularly difficult because they have been manipulated since birth and because it is a natural defense mechanism for children to blame themselves rather than see their parents as selfish, cruel, or unloving.

4. Narcissistic Abuse Is Written in the Body

Particularly for people who have grown up in narcissistic homes, trauma resulting from narcissistic abuse causes not just emotional but physiological long-term damage. According to the American Academy of Pediatrics, "disruption[s] [to] the parent-child relationship are significantly associated with many leading causes of adult death, such as stroke, cancer, and heart disease, and with heavy health service utilization."[4]

As we have discussed, such children experience brain and hormonal trauma responses that can last a lifetime and lead to a variety of acute and chronic dysregulation and disease. They commonly develop CPTSD and other health fallout, including autoimmune disorders, profound sleep disturbance, vulnerability to addiction, self-destructive behavior, and an inclination toward further victimization in their relationships.[5]

5. Narcissistic Abuse Violates Common Codes of Conduct

All societies are held together by codes of conduct. Most of us try to treat others as we wish to be treated. But narcissistically disordered people live by inequity and double standards. When narcissists fall, they not only demand help up but furthermore blame the other person for their fall: *You tripped me! I couldn't see where I was going because you were in the way! I was distracted because you were talking too much! You wanted me to fall!*

6. Narcissistic Abuse Is Supported by Power Structures

Narcissists exploit external systems of power to cover, protect, justify, and enforce what they do. Narcissistic parents have power over their children, narcissistic men over women, narcissistic bosses over employees, narcissistic clerics over congregations, narcissistic teachers over students, narcissistic politicians over communities and societies, and the list goes on. Thus, those targeted face further victimization by the institutions supporting narcissists.

So, if you're feeling impatient with yourself, remember the brutal and insidious nature of NPD and just how devastating narcissistic abuse and its consequences are.

FACING REALITY

As you move out of denial and face the stark facts about what you've been through, one of your biggest challenges is to remain clear about the realities of narcissism so you can let go of unrealistic expectations about the narcissist. Whether you're an adult child, partner, or other family member, perhaps the most difficult thing to accept is that narcissists do not and will never love you as most of us hope to be loved.

Narcissists may say they love you and even believe it. They may for a time put you on a pedestal and treat you like royalty. After they have shown their cruelty, they may at times appear remorseful and make promises to change. They may under certain circumstances behave benignly, even generously. But, as we have learned, with NPD what appears fleetingly to be love is not trustworthy. It is not stable, reciprocal, accepting, selfless, or truly intimate. It is at best idealization, which if it hasn't already will likely crash and burn into a pattern of disappointment, mounting criticism and rage, serial abuse, and possible abandonment, no matter how high you were elevated and how special you felt.

People with NPD *can't love*. Developmentally stunted as young children, they did not learn to accept and love themselves and ultimately despise any club that would have them as a member. When they feel threatened, which is their default state, you become an object to them, not *a someone*, and they feel justified in treating you with scorn and bringing you to your knees.

UNDERSTANDING YOUR GRIEF

As someone processing narcissistic abuse trauma, you are experiencing profound grief. You are grieving a kind of death—in fact, several deaths. There is the death of your belief or hope about the narcissist in your life, the death of who you were in relationship to that person, and the death of what you might have had together but didn't: the healthy relationship, the healthy childhood, the healthy family.

The Partner's Grief

For partners, the grief is about a relationship or marriage and perhaps a family. It is the things you hoped for from or believed about your partner that you now understand to be impossible and/or false. You mourn for the life you made together, the time you shared, what can never be, and what in many ways never was. You also mourn for yourself—who you were with that person, your love and time, your hopes and dreams, the hurt you have gone through, and who you will be in the future with or without that person. And if you have children, you grieve for them. You grieve for their pain, you remember the ways you tried to protect and help them but couldn't, and you mourn for the family that suffered and may continue to suffer now. You grieve the love you might have shared, the family you might have had, the partner and parent you might have been.

The Adult Child's Grief

For the adult child, the first "death" is that of who you needed, hoped, and (more or less) believed your parent (or parents) to be. It is the figurative death of your primary caretaker and model, the person who gave you life and shaped who you are, for better and worse. It is the loss of who s/he could not and will never be. You also mourn for yourself as a child and your childhood itself. You feel that child's confusion and fear, that child's pain and damage, and that child's struggle to survive under brutalizing circumstances. You grieve the ways that child's suffering continues now in adulthood, what it means for your relationships and perhaps family now, and what it means for your future. You grieve the person you might have been and what you might have achieved if you had gotten the stability and nurturance you needed. You mourn the childhood you did not have, your damaged family, and the relationships you might have had with your siblings and perhaps your other parent.

You may be experiencing the double whammy of grief as an adult child of a narcissistic family and as a partner in a narcissistic relationship and maybe family. This is not uncommon, since as we have discussed many people who grow up in such families repeat the pattern in adult relationships.

FEELING YOUR GRIEF

Opening up emotionally to your own grief, especially when it has been buried for a long time, is an intensely painful but crucial step in the recovery process. It can be tempting to focus instead on your cognitive understanding, but cognitive awareness of trauma is not enough. As Karyl McBride explains, you must experience your feelings:

Sit with those feelings. Sit with the pain. . . .

Don't try to talk yourself out of it. Others around you may try to do this. No one wants to see you hurt, and your loved ones may not understand how important this is, so don't listen to them. Let yourself feel![6]

STATES OF GRIEF

Your experience of grief may look like the familiar stages identified by Elisabeth Kübler-Ross in her 1969 book *On Death and Dying*: denial, anger, bargaining, depression, acceptance. Although these stages are often applied to the emotional experience we go through after a loved one dies, in fact Kübler-Ross originally identified them as the emotions we experience about our own death when faced with terminal illness.[7] The other broad misconception about Kübler-Ross's stages of grief is that there is a right order and process that should be followed. In fact, the "stages" are states of mind on the way toward greater acceptance that jump around and don't proceed in order:

There is no straight path or progression of emotions that mourners follow. There is no timeline. Grief is unpredictable, with good days and bad days. We never "get over" the loss of a loved one. Each individual and each loss will have its own unique process for healing.[8]

As you process the losses you've experienced about the narcissist(s) in your life, these states of grief can be helpful guideposts in understanding your feelings.

Denial

This is a natural and often immediate experience after loss. Denial, like shock, is a survival mechanism that gives us time to handle trauma without being completely overwhelmed by the full reality of it. The denial may be numbness, narrowed focus, dissociation, forgetfulness, or a rearrangement of information. Denial can be helpful in the shorter term, but eventually it must be overcome to move forward with healing, particularly to move beyond an abusive relationship with a parent or partner. When we emerge from denial, it can feel disorienting, but our ability to face the facts beyond the denial stage is a necessary step toward overcoming trauma.

Anger

Anger typically follows at some point after loss, especially for a person treated to abuse. But because you have experienced vulnerability, harm, and most likely blame for the abuse you've endured, you may have submerged your anger in numbing or self-destructive patterns. Women in particular may feel discomfort with their own anger. Acknowledging the rightful anger you feel toward the narcissist will help you release the blame, discharge the hurt, and take better care of yourself on your path to recovery.

Bargaining

Bargaining can take different forms. You may try to bargain with the past, with yourself, or with the narcissist. You may tell yourself that if you had acted differently or been a different person, the narcissist would have loved you. Perhaps you think if you change certain things about yourself the conflict will end or you will get the validation you hope for. You may try to get the narcissist or other family members to listen to reason or take responsibility. Bargaining is understandable. But, as we have discussed, the narcissist in your life in all likelihood will not give you validation, will not change, will not be reasonable, and will not take responsibility. The only bargain you can rely on is the change you make in your own life for and about you.

Depression

You've probably been feeling depressed on and off for a long time. It is virtually inevitable to feel depressed around a narcissist and also once you have faced the facts of the disorder and your experiences with it. As you process what you've been through it is normal to feel depressed and at times even defeated and helpless. You may feel less energetic and less social and perhaps lack motivation. But depression does not have to be your fate. As you move toward greater understanding and acceptance, your depressed feelings will lift, your mood will stabilize, and you will feel more energetic and motivated.

Acceptance

Acceptance is not resigning yourself to misery, nor does it mean the pain is erased. At first acceptance may come in spurts interrupted by a return to early forms of grief, such as anger or depression. But in time as you work through your grief, acceptance will increasingly become the norm. Acceptance means you're moving away from hurt; releasing denial, anger, bargaining, and depression; and letting in new relationships, experiences, pleasures, and joys.

Anxiety: The "Missing" State of Grief

In her 2018 book *Anxiety: The Missing Stage of Grief*, Claire Bidwell Smith explores the persistent role of anxiety in the grief process and argues well for its recognition along with the states of grief identified by Kübler-Ross. Although Bidwell Smith is talking about grief from loss, her ideas also apply to losses associated with trauma. Anxiety is a state of agitation or distress that comes from fear—conscious or unconscious fear. Anxiety plays a prominent, ongoing role in the lives of the narcissist's family members. The typical hyperarousal experienced by partners and children is a state of chronic anxiety. As we have discussed, prolonged anxiety wreaks emotional and physical havoc on the body:

> Our fear-response system involves several brain and body systems that send messages that are transmitted over nerve pathways throughout our entire body, using a vast assortment of hormones, proteins, and other neuroendocrine substances. When you encounter a situation that stimulates the fear response, your entire body sends an alarm that prepares you to face the danger or choose to flee. We do not even have to be actively thinking about these fears on a conscious level for them to impact our level of anxiety.[9]

As you process the trauma you've experienced from narcissistic abuse, anxiety will inevitably present itself and recur as you move through the different states of grief. Indeed, anxiety may be your default state, a trauma response that was established a long time ago. Anxiety has a way of begetting more anxiety and can become counterproductive and addictive if it is not accompanied by awareness and action. As Bidwell Smith explains,

Worrying about something can make a person feel as though they are doing something proactive about their specific fear, when really they are just perpetuating a heightened state of alert that keeps them in an anxious state.[10]

In a very real sense everything you are doing to bring awareness to your life, work through your traumatic experience, and embrace healthier states of being is addressing your anxiety. As you release fear and pain and open yourself to healing, your anxiety will diminish. But it may be necessary to consciously treat the anxiety itself, too, through such methods as

- regular exercise,
- mindfulness,
- meditation,
- belly-breathing relaxation,
- yoga, and/or
- medication.

As you reassess the past and face the dysfunction you've experienced, you are processing great loss. You may have cycled through some or all of the states of grief, with sticking points. Perhaps you're stuck on anger or bargaining and wonder whether you'll ever get to acceptance, or you've found yourself in denial about one parent and acceptance about another. You have probably felt moments of each emotion reading this book. Remember that the process is ongoing and may continue to some extent throughout your life, particularly if you grew up in a narcissistic family. But as you consciously work to understand and bring positive change to your life, you are moving into a more stable and peaceful state of acceptance. Acceptance doesn't mean the pain and loss will go away, but it does represent a more functional state of coexistence with the pain and an opening toward better things: less drama, healthier relationships, increased energy, and more hope, humor, and happiness.

REASSESSING YOUR STORIES

Humans are natural storytellers, even those who don't think they are. Stories help us understand the world, make meaning out of our experience, connect us with the past and future, and organize our thoughts and feelings. Stories teach us lessons, inspire and motivate, and serve as cautionary tales. We all have stories about ourselves and our lives. The stories we tell about ourselves say a lot about what we feel and believe, including our unconscious beliefs. Often what we leave out of our stories can tell us as much as what we put in them. And the stories we tell ourselves may be quite different from ones we share with others.

Sometimes we get stuck in our stories. They can become so large and repeated so often that we enshrine them as a fixed part of our personal or family mythology. But our stories may be highly subjective and influenced by many things, such as photographs, things our family members told us and things they didn't tell us, our age when the events happened, and other people's stories. There is also always a context to our stories, which may or may not be represented in our tellings. Context can be where we were, who we were with, our state of mind, the time of year, how old we were, what else was going on in our life, and so forth.

Consider what stories you tell about yourself as a younger person, such as what kind of baby or child you were, how you acted with your siblings and your parents, what you were like socially or in school, what you liked and disliked, what "bad" things you did and what "good" things you did. Then as you consider your stories, ask yourself what evidence you have for them:

1. How do I know this?
2. What do I know that supports or contradicts this?
3. Does it add up and feel true to me?
4. If it doesn't add up, how doesn't it?
5. How does this story make me feel?
6. If this story makes me uncomfortable or upset, why?
7. What underlying assumptions and beliefs does this story reflect?
8. Do I need to reexamine and perhaps change this story?
9. Is there a different story that needs to be told now?

Often our stories need to change to reflect new understandings, uncovered information, and changing emotional truths. As someone dealing with narcissistic abuse trauma, taking a close look at the stories that frame your identity, your partner, and/or your family is vitally important as you work to understand and heal. This is because so much of what narcissists tell us about everything and everyone is distorted or false. Narcissists by nature are *unreliable narrators.* Their selfishness, need to blame others, compulsive projecting, inflated entitlement, lack of self-awareness, hyperdefensiveness, and cognitive distortions inevitably cast reasonable doubt over anything that comes out of their mouth. Their stories should not ever define who other people are, and yet so often they do come to define their family members. Particularly for children of narcissists, reassessing and revising the stories they grew up with is an absolute necessity to healing:

> One of the most important parts of this work comes when we allow our story to change, when we can dig deep enough to recognize that we are not always telling the story that best serves our healing process.[11]

When we get stuck on or find ourselves frequently repeating a particular story or set of details, it may mean we are trying to figure out something important that feels out of reach. Often the parts of a story that make us confused or emotional are sources of fear, guilt, or shame that we need to unpack and look at. It can feel scary, but most often the bad feelings we have carried for years about a story are worse than the reality of the events. Sometimes we uncover upsetting things we have repressed. If this happens, it is probably because we are finally ready to handle what happened and need to look at it so it doesn't continue to have power over us.

As you examine your stories—their surface and hidden meanings and their significance to you now—consider whether they continue to have a place in your life. Consciously owning, updating, or tossing out our stories is a normal and necessary part of growing up that can be extremely freeing and validating.[12]

PANTS ON FIRE

After having her own kids, Rachel unearthed a deep shame she had carried from early childhood. Her narcissistic mother had often said she was a "woeful child" because she was born on a Wednesday, based on an old nursery rhyme.

Deciding to investigate her mother's story, Rachel discovered that she had been born on a *Tuesday*, and her brother, the family golden child and her mother's "absolute favorite," had been born on a Wednesday. <<

ADULT CHILDREN ENDING THE CYCLE

A way of thinking about your own narcissistic trauma is as a disintegration of yourself. Children in narcissistic homes experience assaults to their integrity, or wholeness—the ways their full humanity comes together to support their own healthy development. When we are under assault, we crack and divide, perhaps shut down. We develop more in some places and less in others. Like trees, we root and grow toward water and light wherever we can. Sometimes parasites and disease breach our bark, knots and burls form, and branches break, but we keep moving toward sustaining water and light.

We all have the capacity to learn and grow throughout our lives, but until we learn certain lessons we tend to repeat patterns. If you were raised in a narcissistic home, you are predisposed to fall into similar codependent dynamics in your adult relationships. You are likely to find yourself working for, hiring, befriending, and/or dating or marrying other people from dysfunctional homes. Narcissistic relational dynamics are your normal, something your parents modeled and taught you that you deserve, even if it feels wrong, painful, crazy, dangerous. It is a wound that needs healing.[13]

Breaking the Family Legacy

Having grown up in a narcissistic home, you will find identifying narcissistic behavior in others to be at once more difficult and easier. You are vulnerable to slipping into familiar patterns and ways of thinking about yourself that were ingrained in you from day one. These tendencies may be hardwired into your neurobiological development.[14] But with analysis, education, mindfulness, and proper therapeutic help, you will learn to recognize the signs of narcissism and narcissistic abuse and build the self-esteem to walk away from repeating narcissistic relationships with partners, friends, bosses, therapists, pastors, teachers, and others in your life. You will find your way to self-respect, commit to kindness and justice for yourself and others, and welcome in healthier forms of intimacy in your life. And, perhaps most important, if you have children, you will break the cycle with them, sparing them your suffering and ending what is often a devastating generational pathology. Becoming a parent is often the life experience that initiates a reassessment of how we have been parented and ushers in change.

ADULT CHILDREN AS PARENTS

However you were defined growing up, whether it was as the scapegoat or golden child, hero or lost child, mascot or some complicated hybrid, understanding your role in your family of origin is essential to breaking the cycle with your own children. For many adult children of narcissists, becoming a parent is a pivotal time that can be highly triggering but also potentially liberating and healing.

Through conscious and unconscious associations and memories, parents typically relive their past to some degree according to the ages of their children. As a child begins to talk, starts school, or enters adolescence, for example, parents have associations with their own corresponding experiences at those ages. This is a normal pattern, but for adult children of narcissists (ACoNs), it is fraught with the scarring effects of trauma. When unprocessed trauma resurfaces it can be dislocating and frightening and lead to anguish, anger, disgust, and bewilderment at the ways in which our parents failed to support us. As parents, ACoNs who have not gained an awareness of their family's dysfunction may unwittingly replicate similar patterns in their new families, treating their children to the destructive dynamics they grew up with.

Working on self-awareness at this time is difficult because of the demands of parenting, but it is all the more important precisely because of those demands. Adult children who are able to gain enough self-understanding can use these experiences as opportunities to put the past in perspective and heal old wounds while making things better for their own children. As a parent, you have the opportunity to achieve profound healing through giving to your kids the kind of unconditional love and caretaking you never received enough of yourself.

Remember to be kind to yourself at this time of your life. Being a perfect parent is both impossible and unnecessary. Aim for being a good-enough parent. What your children need is to be seen, loved, and supported for whoever they are, just as you need that and we all need that. Have faith in their ability to do most of the rest of the work of growing up.

REASSESSING THE "GOOD" PARENT

Felix grew up with a domineering, hypercritical father. For decades, he saw his mother as the "good" parent despite the fact that she was self-involved and low on empathy. It wasn't until Felix had his own child and saw how his mother acted with her that he began to acknowledge her failings. "I had always blamed myself for the emptiness and anger I felt about my mother," he said. His view of things shifted when his daughter began to express herself and his mother treated her the same way she had treated him—at times ignoring her needs, resenting her if she didn't automatically comply, becoming frustrated when she asked questions, and avoiding time alone with her. "Mom always portrayed herself as a very caring mother, and compared to my father, she was. But when I saw her with her granddaughter, there was a huge disconnect between what she said about herself and how she acted. I couldn't believe that my mother behaved this way with my daughter, until it finally sank in that it wasn't about my daughter or about me. It was about my mother's limitations, and any child would have received the same treatment," Felix said. "As painful as it was to watch her relationship with my daughter, it was freeing for me to finally see that my mother's inability to connect with me was not because I was unlovable." «

THE ROLE OF THERAPY: REWARDS, RISKS, AND WHAT TO LOOK FOR IN A THERAPIST

For narcissistic abuse trauma sufferers, the right therapy has a big role to play in the recovery process. If we are ready to do the work, a skilled and caring therapist can help us make sense of what we've been through, recognize how the parenting we received shapes our self-beliefs and choices, develop our emotional literacy, and take concrete steps toward healthier and more fulfilling lives. But while therapy can be life-changing for adult children and partners of narcissists, it can be unproductive, even traumatizing, if the mental health professional is unaware of the realities of NPD and narcissistic domestic abuse. Such clients, especially ACoNs, have a profound need to have their experiences validated, perhaps for the first time in their lives. This need, combined with their vulnerability, self-doubt, habit of self-blame, and desire to please makes it imperative that the therapist have a strong understanding of the complexity of NPD and its impact on families and relationships.

Although awareness of narcissistic abuse trauma is growing, there are those in the mental health field who remain ill-equipped to treat it. Los Angeles–based psychotherapist Fiona Steele shifted her practice to work exclusively with narcissistic abuse trauma survivors because of the high demand for such help. "I'm in awe of how few practitioners understand narcissism," she said. "So many of the clients that come to me have dealt with therapists who don't understand the insidious ways narcissists suck out the life of the people around them."[15] Narcissistic abuse trauma counselor Regina Collins also frequently sees people who have been retraumatized in therapy. "My clients often bring up the fact that they feel crazy because their experiences were questioned or negated outright by clinicians who don't understand the behavior patterns of narcissists," she said.[16]

To help bridge the gap, Dr. Karyl McBride, author of *Will I Ever Be Good Enough?* and *Will I Ever Be Free of You?*, founded a 5-step recovery model for ACoNs and a training program for clinicians working with them. She explained the hazards of inadequate training: "If the therapist does not understand the dynamics of narcissism and its debilitating effects, it is easy for them to encourage the 'get over it already, the past is the past' mentality. When they do this, they are not validating the feelings of the client and the relationship or childhood issues are deeply minimized and discounted."[17] McBride encourages people looking for support to vet their mental health providers to make sure they are conversant with narcissism and related trauma.

Licensed clinical psychologist Sharone Weltfreid advises narcissistic abuse survivors to listen to their intuition when choosing a therapist. "The number one predictor of therapeutic success is feeling comfortable with your therapist and confident that they can help you," she said.[18] She encourages people to ask prospective therapists if they understand NPD and have experience treating narcissistic abuse trauma, as well as if they have specific awareness of common narcissistic patterns such as gaslighting, projecting, and triangulating. She recommends choosing a therapist who will help you examine your family of origin dynamics and also work on specific goals for the present. She encourages people seeking help to look for a balance of compassionate validation and active participation rather than an overly directive approach or overly passive listening approach.

Dr. Weltfreid also emphasized the importance of properly vetting couples therapists, noting that one client of hers had sought help from a couples therapist only to have her narcissistic partner charm the therapist into working alone with him, a scenario often cited by traumatized partners.

Steele pointed out the need, when looking for a qualified therapist, to inquire about treatment toolkits beyond talk therapy. "Processing by talking is important, but it's not enough to engage the body's underlying trauma," she said. Like many clinicians who work with narcissistic abuse trauma survivors, she offers emotional freedom therapy (EFT) and eye movement desensitization and reprocessing therapy (EMDR), which are believed to help the body release the effects of long-held trauma.

It is also essential to vet therapists for narcissistic traits and listen to your instincts if your inner "nardar" is sending you warning signals. The therapeutic relationship rests on compassion, trust, respect, and healthy boundaries. A good therapist recognizes your vulnerability, honors your need for safety, and supports your process of building self-awareness and self-esteem. A therapist who displays poor listening, boundary violations, and/or a judgmental response is not worthy of your trust. If you find yourself in such a relationship, walk away and consider the experience a lesson learned.

Questions to Ask When Looking for a Therapist

1. What is your experience with NPD?
2. What is your experience with narcissistic abuse trauma?
3. Do you explore family-of-origin dynamics?
4. Do you establish and work toward concrete goals?

Look for a therapist who:

1. provides active listening
2. displays compassion
3. validates your feelings
4. models good boundaries
5. displays honesty and directness
6. can laugh at themselves

7. identifies your self-defeating patterns
8. provides a vocabulary for feelings
9. gives homework if you want it
10. offers flexible approaches
11. gives feedback
12. is receptive to feedback

Avoid a therapist who:

1. displays impatience or arrogance
2. has rigid or weak boundaries
3. is dismissive
4. is defensive
5. has a judgmental or authoritarian attitude
6. is emotionally detached
7. makes sweeping statements
8. draws conclusions too quickly
9. dismisses your need for limited or no contact with the narcissist
10. uses a rigid methodology
11. shows a lack of interest or curiosity
12. frequently relates things back to him-/herself
13. is easily manipulated
14. doesn't give feedback
15. shuts down or rejects feedback
16. is overly serious or humorless

twenty

Managing the Narcissist in Your Life

A S YOU GAIN PERSPECTIVE ABOUT NARCISSISM AND ITS EFFECT ON YOU, you may still be tied to the narcissist in one way or another, as a partner, coparenting ex, parent, or other family member. Here are some strategies for managing such relationships, while protecting yourself.

WHEN THE NARCISSIST IS NICE

One of the most disorienting things about narcissists is that they can be nice. If they are feeling adequately attended to and not threatened, they can be fun and likeable, even charming. Under the right circumstances, narcissists may be interested, affectionate, playful, funny, helpful, generous, thoughtful, even insightful, particularly if it reinforces a belief about themselves that they feel good about, such as "I am a wonderful mother/father." Although people with NPD have a crippling mental condition, in their most secure moments they may even step beyond their defenses and perhaps see things outside their immediate perspective. For example, narcissists might, perhaps for the first time,

- tell their child that they are proud of them,
- admit that they should have been less self-involved as a parent,
- admit to their spouse that they were right about something they had previously fought about,

- agree to family or marriage counseling,
- show spontaneous affection,
- acknowledge an adult child's accomplishments or success, or
- tell their spouse that s/he is a good partner or parent.

The problem is that narcissists' "nice" overtures can be difficult, even impossible to discern from their manipulations. If you are the recipient of narcissists' apparent kindness, particularly if you have known them for a while, you will be rightfully confused by the turnabout. You may wonder whether the gesture is sincere or yet another tactical maneuver to hoover you back in or otherwise set you up for further manipulation or an ambush. You may find yourself doubting what you've come to understand about them and wonder whether you misjudged them. The narcissists themselves probably do not fully understand their own feelings or motives or how long they may last. It is important to keep in mind that people with NPD give when it is in some way validating for them and fits with an image they have of themselves, not selflessly because they are emotionally attuned and have someone else's best interests at heart.

Accept the Good, with Healthy Skepticism

If a narcissist's affection feels real, try to accept it at face value and feel good about that long-craved-for affirmation. It may be one of only a handful of moments or even the first of its kind in the relationship. But as a veteran of the narcissist's abuse, you also should remain skeptical of authentic lasting growth in the narcissist, something that at best will be very limited. Perhaps most important, do not base conclusions or decisions upon what may be a temporary shift or opening. You would be wise not to push the issue by pulling out a laundry list of complaints or suddenly confiding things long held in check. If you are an adult child of a narcissist, you may be tempted to resume or increase contact, but you should instead let the dust settle to consider the situation and see what happens next. The same goes if you are an ex, sibling, or friend who is tempted to reconcile with a narcissist. Enjoy the moment, even savor it, but for your mental and physical well-being remember the bigger picture and keep your expectations in check.

ASSERTING BOUNDARIES

Even for the most secure adults from healthy and loving families, it can be difficult to break away from parental influence, both direct and indirect, and establish adult independence. If you're an adult child of narcissists (ACoN), finding stable footing and establishing healthy boundaries is a lifelong struggle.

As we have discussed, boundaries are always disrupted in narcissistic homes. Narcissists' intense neediness, distorted and vacillating self-concept, and lack of emotional empathy drive them to exploit their children at the expense of their children's needs. Such parents disregard their children's boundaries because they view their kids as manipulatable extensions of themselves, not as individuals with their own unique personality, passions, and needs to be acknowledged and respected. As we have discussed, children in such circumstances experience boundary violations that can include neglect, outright abuse, parentification, engulfment, infantilization, and/or idealization/overvaluation.

As an ACoN, you probably struggle to balance your need for independence with your desire for intimacy. You may find it difficult to identify your feelings and needs and separate them from those of others. Possibly you tend toward people-pleasing and excessive caregiving, compulsively placing the needs of others before your own. You may be highly self-protective and tend to distrust others, or you may rush to intimacy and lose yourself in relationships. You may have distorted ideas about how important or influential (too much or too little) you are to other people. You probably carry a heavy weight of (false) responsibility and (undeserved) guilt, and as a result you may feel complexly entangled with and at the same time estranged from your family members.

 ARE YOU MY MOTHER?

At 45, Molly is well aware of her mother's cruelty, which has included abetting her father's and brother's physical and sexual abuse of Molly, as well as a lifetime of emotional neglect. Molly has been through years of therapy and participates regularly in online support groups for children of narcissists. She said, "I know I have a conscious denial about my mother. I'm still looking for love from her. When I tell her I love her, I'm thinking, 'Damn it, I want you to love me back!'" Seeing how much her mother hurts Molly, Molly's husband wants her to cut off contact. "It takes him three days to put me together again after I see or speak with my mother," Molly said. "But I'm just not ready to walk away from the relationship. I know it's not rational, but she's my mother." ‹‹

Making matters more painful, as a child you were probably deeply invested in "winning" your parents' love as opposed to getting it unconditionally, an ingrained compulsion that you may still feel as an adult. All children want and need their parents to love them, and for ACoNs that empty feeling tends to persist a very long time. Even realizing your parents are narcissistic and understanding NPD does not make it easy to let go of the fantasy that they will someday finally take responsibility for their egregious actions and provide appropriate love and care. Nor does it make setting boundaries with them easy. Narcissistic parents strongly resist their adult children's attempts to assert appropriate boundaries because boundaries threaten their ability to control their image to the world and their domineering hold on the family.

Strategies for Setting Healthy Boundaries

Having had your boundaries crossed your whole life in a variety of ways, you are likely to struggle to define what "normal" healthy boundaries are in your other relationships, including those with your partner and, if you have them, children. Sometimes the worst models in life teach the most important lessons, and not repeating your parents' abuses and manipulations can be your best guide. Paying attention to and respecting your own needs and feelings is crucial to setting appropriate boundaries in all areas of life. It is also good modeling for your children. Boundaries show us where we and others begin and end, what is needed and not needed, and what is allowed and not allowed. They are flexible enough to enable us to connect with others while being defined and strong enough to support our own healthy individual identity and comfort zone.

Here are ways to help set and sustain good boundaries in your life:

1. Tune In to Your Feelings

Listen to yourself. Practice introspection. The more you practice attuning with your feelings and exploring what they mean, the better you'll get at it. If you feel anxious, afraid, or resentful, for example, it may indicate that someone is violating your boundaries. Similarly, if you are procrastinating or ignoring something, it may be because you feel your boundaries are threatened. Keeping a journal, taking time for deep breathing, or talking with a trusted friend can help make you more aware of your feelings.

2. Give Yourself Permission to Say No

Although you may not have had permission to say no to your parents, healthy people say no and accept no in stride and without guilt or resentment. No lets other people know what you are comfortable doing or not doing and what you are comfortable with them doing or not doing. As an adult you need to accept the important role of no in your life and learn to assert it with your parents for your own emotional well-being. If you have children, part of your job as a loving and responsive parent is to set appropriate and safe limits for your kids, which includes saying no. It does not have to be harsh or punishing, and it can be delivered in a neutral, loving, or humorous way. Provided it is affectionate, the more humor the better! Strive for a balance between no and yes.

3. Caretake Yourself

Children of narcissists are conditioned to take care of their parents in various ways, often at their own expense. Even if you did not do much direct caretaking of your parents and even if they told you that *everything was for you*, they inevitably communicated the message that your needs were a distant second to theirs. We all have needs that do not go away, and as an adult, now it is your job to work on meeting those needs. Part of maintaining healthy boundaries is recognizing and respecting your need for self-care. That means taking time for yourself, practicing healthy habits, relaxing, and making time for fun.

4. Reach Out

ACoNs have been trained to internalize blame and keep family affairs private, and they often isolate themselves as a result. Setting healthy boundaries doesn't just mean saying no. It can also mean opening yourself to new experiences and saying yes to getting closer to people who are trustworthy.

5. Seek Safe Support

ACoNs learn to ignore their own feelings and needs in service of the narcissistic parent's demands. Unburying your feelings with a trusted counselor and with people who understand is essential for processing the trauma of the past and moving beyond it. Note that it is vital to find a therapist or coach conversant with narcissism, since those who are not can unwittingly invalidate your feelings and experiences and trigger old trauma. The same is true for pastors, friends, and other members of your social circle. Confiding in others who do not understand narcissism can backfire, leading to misunderstandings, judgment, and ill-advised suggestions.

6. Be Direct

It is not easy for ACoNs, but being direct about your boundaries—what you do and don't want and will and won't do—is an important part of being a functional adult. Becoming direct about your needs and limits may feel awkward at first, but it will get easier with practice. Directness with narcissists is another matter, however, and it may be wiser to set boundaries without telling them what you are doing or why. If anyone has earned the path of least resistance, it's you.

7. Understand Your Responsibilities

Since you have been burdened with responsibility for your demanding narcissistic parent and/or made to feel helpless and dependent on that parent, you probably have a distorted sense of how much responsibility you do and don't have. Here are some guidelines:

You are *not* responsible for

- your parent's self-esteem,
- your parent's happiness,
- your parent's relationships,
- your parent's treatment of you,
- your parent's treatment of others,
- your parent's inappropriate and embarrassing behavior,
- your parent's reputation with others,
- your parent's expectations,

- your other family members' happiness, and
- your other family members' treatment of you.

You *are* responsible for
- how you react to your parent,
- how you react to your other family members,
- maintaining boundaries with your parent and other family members,
- managing your expectations,
- your choices,
- your relationships,
- your health,
- your attitude,
- your behavior in your family, and
- getting your needs met.

 BODY BOUNDARIES

Oscar grew up with a mother and father who routinely ignored his need for physical boundaries, including taking showers with him until he finally refused to at age 10. With his own son, he wanted to have better boundaries, but at times wasn't sure what that should look like. When his son was 7, he began to be shy about being naked around Oscar. "At first I was confused and wondered whether something was wrong. But when my son told me he wanted privacy, I realized it was healthy and I was happy to honor that," he said. ‹‹

Protecting Yourself Legally

With narcissistic parents or family members, you may be vulnerable legally. Narcissists feel above the law and frequently manipulate and/or violate rules, laws, and legal systems to their benefit or to spite others. It's important not to be naive about how quickly and badly situations can spin out of control. Are you and your partner, kids, animal companions, home, car, and other valuables safe and legally in your hands? Is your same-sex or otherwise unmarried relationship secure? If something happens to you, do you know if your loved ones will have access to you in the hospital, the right to make decisions on your behalf, and full ownership of your shared kids, pets, home, and possessions? Are your wishes spelled out in your will?

If your parents or other family members are harassing you, lying about you, falsely accusing you, or otherwise threatening or violating your safety, have you documented the abuse? It may be necessary to record or take screen shots of interactions, write down dates and details, and get witnesses for corroboration. If you have any concerns, seek legal advice. Domestic violence services in your city, county, or state may provide free information and legal consultation, so make sure to avail yourself of their services if you need the support.

Going Limited or No Contact

As an ACoN, you have been groomed to play a particular role in the narcissistic family system. Unless your parents get help and want to change, they will never stop pushing you to continue playing that role, or other ones that suit the moment, because as far as they are concerned it is your life purpose. Your siblings and other relatives also may push you to continue the role cast for you in childhood. Depending on their own level of awareness and investment in the existing family structure, they may or may not respect your need to set boundaries. They may continue to target you as the family scapegoat or resent you for your "privilege" as the golden child. They may expect you to continue as selfless caretaker to your parents, heroic problem solver, acquiescent sidekick, or clowning comedian. If they resist your efforts to change, you may find yourself having to make difficult decisions about how much to allow them into your life as you work toward a healthy distance from the dysfunction and pain in your family of origin.

As an ACoN, you are confronting the reality that your parent or parents cannot reciprocate all but the most primitive form of love, far from the unconditional love we all hope to give and receive within our families. In some cases, limited or no contact with your parents may be your only way to avoid conflict and further harm. You may need to reduce or block their social media, phone, and text access. If your family is actively abusive, going no contact is probably your healthiest and safest choice, at least for a period of time.

Others may regard your decision to go no contact with your parents and/or family as extreme and unreasonable and may attempt to change your mind. Family members may try to hoover you back in the fold using guilt, drama, or carrots like financial help. It is not above some narcissists to exaggerate or altogether feign illness to garner attention and sympathy. Others who are somehow invested in helping maintain the dysfunctional status quo or simply don't understand the realities you are dealing with also may try to interfere. Keep in mind that very few people cut out family members frivolously. Most children, including adult children, are more apt to blame themselves than their parents for problems in the relationship, often remaining loyal beyond all reason. Denial and self-blame are, as we know, the first line of defense for the child with abusive parents. For adult children of narcissists, going no contact is typically an ambivalent, painful, and last-ditch option necessary for safety and sanity. The choice to go no contact is yours, and it is not your job to explain or justify to anyone your reasons for doing so. It is often easiest to keep your no-contact status on a need-to-know basis with people in your life. You may want to rehearse a simple response you can use with others if your no-contact status comes up.

When setting boundaries with your family of origin, if you have a family of your own you need to consider the stakes for them as well as for yourself. In particular, you need to help your children navigate away from the narcissistic family legacy of emotional and physical trauma.

WHAT TO EXPECT FROM THE AGING NARCISSIST

Aging is hard. For so many of us, losing our vitality and facing our mortality is a scary, painful experience. But we discover upsides, like the satisfactions of earned competency, long-term connections with family and friends, recognizing our core values and releasing shallow pursuits, reaping the fruits of our professional and personal labors, and seeing our kids and grandkids thrive and helping them when they falter. We become more patient, present, and grateful for life's pleasures. The wise among us take time to listen, reflect, savor, and continue finding ways to grow and give back, like deeply ringed trees breathing out life-giving oxygen.

Sadly, people with NPD tend not to age well. Instead of maturing, mellowing, and gaining wisdom, narcissists, unless helped with treatment, remain emotionally impaired children whose deficient empathy and self-centered neediness often intensify with aging. They are apt to view growing old as a series of ravaging defeats that they struggle against with denial, defiance, resentment, and/or depressed resignation.

Bitterness

Having relied heavily on such externalities as their looks, physical strength, connections, or professional achievement to fortify their fragile self-esteem, older narcissists find themselves increasingly stripped of their defenses and diminished in their ability to charm, influence, impress, control, and otherwise exert power over others. Since they rarely feel satisfied or take responsibility for their actions or circumstances, they are inclined to grow bitter and feel victimized by life, blaming others and cruel fate for their disappointments.

People with NPD tend to age into more extreme versions of their most defensive selves. And when dementia comes into the picture, it can exacerbate matters. Aging narcissists may become more

- desperate,
- deluded,
- paranoid,
- cynical,
- irrational,
- bitter,
- blaming,
- intolerant,
- angry,
- rigid, and
- mean.

Isolation

Because of narcissists' lack of compassion and their antagonism, as they age, their family relationships and friendships often falter or fail, leaving them lonely and isolated:

- Spouses may have left or withdrawn to avoid their criticism and combativeness.
- Adult children may have pulled away or cut contact altogether because of their toxic influence.
- Grandchildren may be estranged from them because the narcissist's adult children have asserted boundaries to protect their kids.
- Friends may have pulled away because of the narcissist's unmasked arrogance, selfishness, and envy.
- Neighbors and other community members may have rejected them because of their callous behavior and rude assertions of superiority and entitlement.
- Extended family may have excluded them because of their divisiveness.

Bigotry

As their personal power fades and their social sphere narrows, narcissists are more likely to look for scapegoats anywhere they can. Their increasingly desperate grandiose delusions often bring out bigotry and assertions of superiority over marginalized people, including other old people. Often older narcissists are disgusted by others their own age, seeing themselves as more attractive, youthful, and sharp-minded than their peers. Aging narcissists also may express sexism, homophobia, and racism to bolster themselves against their feelings of lost power over others.

 FOREVER YOUNG

Morgan loved going to the gym and prided herself on looking young for her age, with help from numerous plastic surgeries. As she grew older, she became haughty with people her own age, whom she regarded as "pathetic, boring, and ugly." In her community was a center for seniors with many good resources and activities, but Morgan didn't want to associate with old people. Well into her 80s, she believed she could pass for being in her 50s and rejected any men who spoke to her who were older than that. She also rejected women her age, believing they were envious of her and only interested in stealing her things. Although she was very lonely and in need of help, she refused her son's offer to live near him and see more of her grandchildren because she didn't want people to know that she was old enough to be a grandmother. «

TIPS FOR HANDLING AGING NARCISSISTIC PARENTS

Managing aging narcissistic parents is a struggle. They tend to magnify problems by either denying their need for help or playing up their victimhood. They may ignore medical advice and refuse care or exaggerate their needs and make unreasonable drama and demands. They will find it difficult to understand your position as a younger adult who has a full plate of responsibilities, possibly including caring for your own kids at home. Making matters more strained, they may be alienated from family members and others in their social circles.

As with any aging parents, you will need to assess your parents' needs, your own resources, and your own willingness to be involved. Over time their needs will increase, requiring you to periodically reassess things. Whether you help at all may be a difficult choice. Parents who have been actively abusive or violent may not be safe to be around, or there may be too much water under the bridge for you. Also consider your motives for getting involved. Are you hoping to get approval or prove something? Try to be clear with yourself and realistic about your expectations. It is your job to put your needs and those of your current family first.

Here are more tips for managing the situation:

1. **Set boundaries.** Think hard about what you are willing to do and be clear with your parents about your limits. Try not to let feelings of guilt make decisions for you.

2. **Be direct and unemotional.** Try not to react to fawning, baiting, melodrama, or other forms of manipulation. It is better for everyone to keep expectations clear.

3. **Share responsibility.** If you have siblings or other family or family friends able to help, divvy up responsibilities. Be realistic about what you can handle.

4. **Create a schedule.** A schedule can help to provide structure, manage expectations, and stay organized.

5. **Use community resources.** Many communities have free or affordable services for seniors, such as meals, transportation, classes, group outings, and health-related care. Your parents may have free gym membership and other preventative care perks through their health

insurance. If your parents resist community help, preferring that you do it, you will need to make it clear what you will and won't do. When faced with the reality, they may change their mind about accepting outside help.

6. **Allow consequences to play out.** The narcissistic personality is often shielded from consequences by enabling partners and other family members or even codependent friends. But consequences are often the only things that motivate people to change their behavior and take responsibility. Within safe parameters, try to allow natural consequences to occur so that your parents can be in charge of their lives as much as possible. If that means not being together on Thanksgiving, so be it.

7. **Talk to doctors.** You may need to accompany your parents to doctor appointments or find another way to speak with their doctors to get accurate information and/or help them manage their health care and medications.

8. **Step back from drama.** Don't take responsibility for your parents' behavior or reputation with others. How your parents act is their responsibility, not yours. Unless it endangers someone or jeopardizes their care or safety, try not to get involved.

9. **Accept help if it helps.** If your parents can reciprocate your help in certain ways, take the help. But be clear about what the help means for you both. If there are strings attached that are unacceptable, that's a deal breaker.

10. **Walk away from bigotry.** If your parents are expressing sexism, racism, or other forms of bigotry that you find degrading, let them know it's not allowed on your watch.

EXERCISING HEALTHY BOUNDARIES

When Edward lost his driver's license because of his failing vision, he was furious. Other older people in his neighborhood got help from volunteer drivers in the community, but Edward said getting rides from strangers was beneath him and asked his son Bernie to drive him whenever he needed to go anywhere. Bernie, who worked and had a family at home, quickly found himself overwhelmed.

He realized he needed to set limits, so he told his father he would drive him to the grocery store once a week and to doctor appointments, but would not drive him to and from the gym. Angry, Edward said he would quit the gym. "I was tempted to just drive him to the gym because I knew it was his favorite thing to do and I didn't want him to lose that," Bernie said. "But it was too much time for me and he could go if he was willing to accept outside help, so I told him that was his choice. One day of skipping the gym was enough motivation to get Dad to use the volunteer driving service. Now he actually enjoys the company." <<

twenty-one

Steps to Recovery

YOU'VE FIGURED OUT THAT YOUR PARTNER OR EX IS A NARCISSIST AND/OR that one or more of your parents are narcissistic. They may be hard-core with NPD or they may have narcissistic traits. They may be part of a complex collection of parents, stepparents, in-laws, siblings, and other family members who fall in various places along the narcissism and codependency continuum. Whatever the reality is in your relationship or family and however old you are, you need to move forward with your own life. It's never too late or too early to work on your emotional literacy and healing. Even if you are a minor still living at home, there are many ways you can help yourself.

As you work on yourself, remember that healing takes awareness, patience, and practice. At times it calls upon us to sit still, and at other times it demands action. There are always setbacks and periods of discouragement. Feeling lost is often necessary to help you recognize the path you want to be on. Remember also that our thoughts and feelings, physical body and mind are not separate things but are in fact *intrinsically connected*. When we deny, devalue, or neglect one dimension of ourselves, we hurt all dimensions. Embrace every part of yourself, and make getting better your number one priority. There is nothing more important.

HEALING STRATEGIES

Here are practical steps you can take to work on recovery. Some of the strategies listed are aimed at anyone dealing with the aftermath of narcissistic abuse, and some are specifically directed at adult children of narcissists.

Educate Yourself about Narcissism

If you're new to the realization that your partner or one or more of your family members is narcissistic, you need to keep learning about what you're dealing with. Scour the Internet for good resources (see some listed at the end of this book). Read, join chat forums, watch movies and shows with narcissistic characters, and talk with understanding allies. The more you educate yourself and find support, the more you will understand what you've been through and what you need to do to move beyond the toxic influence of your family. Processing the past, particularly a traumatic one that may be spilling into the present, takes time and a lot of repetition.

Seek Professional Help

Opening up and asking for help is difficult for many of us, but ACoNs are especially prone to denying their needs and going it alone. After all, you have most likely been programmed to swallow your feelings, ignore your pain, hide your vulnerabilities, and perhaps give help but seldom ask for it. You also may have been taught that seeking therapy is a form of weakness or self-indulgence. Going it alone may feel safer for you, but long-term trauma is a heavy burden that most of us are not equipped to handle, particularly when it is rooted in childhood. Support from a qualified psychologist or counselor can help you move out of the darkness of silent suffering and self-destruction into the light of self-awareness and positive change. Look for a therapist who understands narcissistic abuse and offers a compassionate, validating, and flexible approach to help you explore your trauma history and work toward concrete goals. See Chapter 19 for more about finding a qualified therapist and avoiding an unqualified one.

Accept That the Narcissist Won't Change

One of the most difficult challenges you face is accepting that the narcissist in your life in all likelihood will not change. If s/he finds a way to make personal progress toward a healthier state of being, great, but you should assume s/he won't. As we have discussed, narcissists rarely change unless through appropriate intensive therapy, which in most cases they do not seek out or stick with. When they are acting nicer, it is usually temporary, conditional, and possibly for manipulative reasons. Expecting that person to finally give you the love you have craved is natural, but it makes you vulnerable to further abuse and keeps you from moving on.

Recognize Your Codependent/Enabling Parent

With a narcissistic parent, you also may have a codependent, enabling one. By going along with and/or excusing the narcissist's abusive behavior enablers essentially normalize and help sustain it. By not naming the abuse and not protecting their kids from it, enabling parents become complicit, even if they are also victimized by it. Those parents may even sustain the family's narcissistic value system by actively perpetrating the abuse. As we discussed in Chapter 13, people who become codependent to a narcissistic partner have more than likely come out of similar home environments with one or more narcissistic or otherwise emotionally demanding and unstable parents. They may not be aware of the parallels between past and present, but they are driven by strong emotional, psychological, and physiological imperatives.

Sometimes forgiving the codependent parent can be as hard as or harder than forgiving the narcissistic parent. People with NPD are impaired with a severe and rigid personality disorder rooted in childhood. Although the narcissist behaves dreadfully, you may find yourself at times feeling worse about the more "functional" parent. You may wonder why that parent excused the narcissist and didn't protect you from abuse, and you may feel betrayed by her/his complicity. On the other hand, talking with that parent about the unhealthy family dynamics and how they hurt you can be healing if s/he is open to what you have to say. Sometimes it is possible to get closer with the other parent and support each other in forming more healthy patterns in your lives.

Recognize Your Family Role

Were you a scapegoat, golden child, hero, mascot, lost child, or somewhere in between? Have you acted at times as a flying monkey? Roles can be fluid in the narcissistic family, depending on changing circumstances and the narcissist's shifting agenda. Perhaps you have been idealized at times and scapegoated at other times. Perhaps you have functioned as a caretaker but have also been ignored and neglected. Are you still operating in the same role with your family members now? Understanding the primary role you played and how that influenced your identity is an important part of building self-awareness and addressing your patterns as an adult.

Seek Allies in Your Family

It is important to remember that you and your family members have been part of a warped system orchestrated by the dominant narcissist to serve her/his needs. You have all been fighting to survive as best you can with the roles you have been cast in. The most powerful defense against the narcissist is a unified front against her/him. If you can find mutual understanding and unity with your other family members, that can be an empowering way to shut down the narcissist's abusive behavior and end hurtful patterns, as well as a profound source of validation and healing for what you have been through. However, if your other parent or siblings are not trustworthy or open to talking about the narcissism in your family, you need above all to protect yourself and limit or perhaps end contact with them.

Assert Boundaries

Because of their dysfunctional conscience and need to control the narrative, narcissists constantly violate boundaries. As a narcissist's child, you have been objectified—not respected as a person with your own identity. As long as you allow it, your parents will try to tell you what you think and feel and insist on your compliance with their distorted version of reality no matter how absurd or harmful. As we have discussed before, one of the most difficult and important things you must do for yourself as a survivor is to establish healthy boundaries with the narcissist and in your own life. Understanding what that means and getting comfortable doing it can take considerable time and practice, but you will get there.

 BOUNDARY BUMPER CARS

With highly manipulative parents, Justine grew up not knowing what healthy boundaries looked like. "I thought if I said no to people they would reject me, so I went along with all kinds of things I didn't want," she said. When she began working on setting boundaries, she found herself swinging to the other extreme. "I really pulled away from people and social situations because I was afraid I would fall into old patterns." But as she became more confident and self-aware, she learned to trust her feelings and find balance. "Now I usually know what I want and feel fine about saying yes or no," she said. "I realize if the other person doesn't like it, that's their issue." <<

Attune to Your Feelings

As the child of a narcissistic parent, you have been systematically trained to ignore your feelings, even to fear and hate them. That parent regards your feelings as a direct threat when they conflict with what s/he needs, believes, and demands. In the narcissistic family, only the narcissist's feelings matter, and everyone else's must be sublimated or silenced through denial, guilt, gaslighting, shame, rage, and the list goes on.

Perhaps the most important thing to do for your healing is to reconnect with your feelings. They are there, and they always have been. Let them in, listen to them, carry them with respect. In your feelings, you will locate yourself and your way through and out of the narcissist's "alternative facts" universe. Alice Miller, in her powerful book on narcissistic trauma *The Drama of the Gifted Child*, puts it this way: "Our feelings will always reveal the true story, which no one else knows and which only we can discover."[1]

Since you have been violated in innumerable ways by your parent, you will have to navigate through intense confusion, hurt, and anger. Most narcissists constantly project their own self-serving motives and emotions onto others and blame others for or even accuse them of their own abusive behavior, so at first you may not know what you really feel versus what you have been conditioned to believe. As you learn to attune to your feelings, be patient. Try not to judge yourself. Feelings are feelings are feelings. They deserve, and in the scheme of things insist upon, recognition and respect.

Recognize Your Triggers

Coming out of a narcissistic family and/or relationship also means you have trauma triggers, or things that set off painful feelings or extreme emotional reactions. Triggers can be particular words, situations, sensory experiences, places, or people. Just being around the narcissist in your life may be trigger enough to elicit and escalate emotions such as fear or anger. Often our triggers feel so overwhelming they make us want to escape into addictive behavior. Especially if they formed early in life, triggers can be unconscious neurological patterns that are difficult to resist. Like well-worn paths, they beckon us to follow them. It may take some bushwhacking, but changing our reactions into thoughtful responses can help us create new pathways that take us to better places. When we become aware of our triggers, we can consciously work to remap our brain and learn healthier ways of thinking, feeling, and acting.

Stop Blaming Yourself

Especially if you've been heavily scapegoated, you are likely to blame yourself automatically and feel guilt for things beyond your control or responsibility. Narcissists are experts at deflecting and projecting blame onto others. If they raged at you and you stood up for yourself, you attacked them. If they hit you, you drove them to it and deserved it. If they are ashamed of their body, you have body issues. One of the best ways to break the unhealthy dynamics is to stop blaming yourself for what was never your responsibility or fault to begin with.

Stop Hurting Yourself

Along with blaming yourself, you may struggle with patterns of poor self-care and self-abuse. As someone raised in a narcissistic family, you are prone to neglectful, risky, controlling, self-punishing, and self-soothing but destructive behaviors, such as

- overexercising,
- disordered eating,
- cutting and other forms of self-harm,
- thrill-seeking,
- ignoring pain,
- not seeking medical help,
- overworking,
- avoidance, and
- compulsive and/or unsafe sex.

Your self-neglect and self-harm are internalizations of the narcissistic abuse you grew up with. By engaging in self-defeating behavior you continue to give the narcissist power over you. You also exacerbate the trauma you have already endured. Patterns of self-harm can be extremely hard to break, so seek support from professionals who understand CPTSD.

Address Your Addictions

Many people who have grown up with trauma and/or experienced it in adulthood fall into addictive patterns. Sitting with pain can feel overwhelming, and efforts to control, numb, or distract ourselves are understandable attempts to cope with suffering and negative emotions. Things like compulsive shopping, gaming, gambling, substance abuse, binge eating, guru addiction, and workaholism can seem to offer relief from such pain by giving us a feel-good shot of dopamine from our brain's reward center. But over time as we develop tolerance, our reward response requires increasing amounts of our drug of choice to make us feel good. One or two drinks are no longer enough so we drink more and more, chasing the "high" that increasingly feels out of reach and poisoning ourselves in the process. As the addiction advances, we come to feel that we can't live—or don't want to—without it, and our "need" for it eclipses all else.

As someone working on self-awareness and personal healing from trauma, you need to be aware of your vulnerability to addiction. If you also have a genetic predisposition (evident in your family) to certain addictions, it is all the more important to work actively on preventing it or taking steps to overcome it. Remember to treat yourself with respect and compassion along the way. Try not to attach shame to it. Addiction *does not* mean you are a "bad," weak, or selfish person. It does not require you "to submit to a higher power" if you do not find that idea helpful. Instead recognize that your addictive behavior is one more way you have tried to manage trauma.

Breaking addiction can be extremely difficult, and depending on your situation you may need to seek out specialized help for it in the form of a therapist, support group, coach, and/or treatment program. It may be impossible to believe right now, but you can reach a place where the addiction no longer dominates your thoughts or exerts power over you. People from all walks of life overcome addictions, and it is powerfully liberating when you get there. You can get there.

Get Physical

We are all physical beings. Even, and perhaps especially, if the narcissist(s) in your life said you were clumsy, nonathletic, lazy, slow, and the like, movement and exercise are important for all aspects of your health. As you process trauma and work on healing, getting your blood flowing and muscles working will help you

- release tension and anxiety,
- clear your mind,
- feel more energetic,
- sleep better,
- digest better,
- reduce pain,
- feel pleasure, and
- feel more confident.

Choose something you like to do that you can sustain regularly. It can be an individual activity, such as walking or biking, or it can be social, such as disc golf or dancing. There are no rules. Make it fun. And if you have a dog, include your canine best friend!

Establish Healthy Routines

Exercising regularly is only one part of an overall healthy and stable pattern in your life. As someone who has experienced trauma, you have had your emotions and health dysregulated and you may have taken on perfectionist, numbing, and/or self-destructive habits that are undermining your well-being. This makes sticking to a healthy routine all the more important now.

- **Set regular times to sleep and wake.** Getting to sleep earlier allows your body to do the restorative work it needs to do. Getting up on the early side keeps us in sync with life's rhythms.
- **Do work you like.** Even if you don't like your job, try to make time to do other forms of work that give you a sense of purpose and accomplishment, such as gardening, making art, building something, taking care of animals or people in need, or even just reading.

- **Stay connected.** Even if you prefer time alone or just with your family, make sure to stay connected with people who matter to you. It will make you happier and give you needed perspective.
- **Spend time in nature.** *Last Child in the Woods: Saving Our Children From Nature-Deficit Disorder* author Richard Louv reminds us how important time outside in nature is for our children's development, health, and happiness,[2] but that also applies to adults. Make time outside. Be with trees. Watch birds. Lie in the grass. Turn on your sensory system to life's music.
- **Spend time with animals.** Animals see us in ways people cannot. And we feel free to be ourselves with them in ways that often feel more authentic than what we show the rest of the world. Kiss your cat.
- **Eat well.** Try to spend time with your food. Food is a fundamental that deserves a place of honor in our lives. Make the experience of preparing and eating food mindful, healthy, and pleasurable. Share it with people you love.
- **Breathe.** This seems obvious, but getting oxygen flowing well in and out of our bodies can be harder than it sounds while being extremely healing. Practice belly-breathing, which involves drawing our breath deep down fully into our lower lungs. Often, especially when we are stressed, we take short shallow breaths that don't oxygenate our body well. Belly-breathing should be relaxed and slow, not forced or gasping, with your belly rising up and down. If you need help, look online for instructions. It takes some mindfulness but quickly becomes natural. The power of good breathing should not be underestimated. You literally can't feel stressed out when you are properly belly-breathing.

REMEMBERING TO BREATHE

When Gino saw a therapist for help with stress, she explained that he was having panic attacks with hyperventilation. This led him to remember something he had buried from childhood. "My father was an angry and violent man, and I felt terrified when he hit my mother and older brother," Gino said. "I would forget to breathe and pass out. Now I practice my breathing every day and catch myself when I start to have trouble." <<

Identify Triggering Times

As you work on establishing your own healthy routines, also consider the routines you experienced growing up. Certain times of day, days of the week, or times of the year may have been particularly stressful. Dinnertime, for example, is often fraught with conflict in the narcissistic family. Mornings getting ready for school are also typical times of stress. If there was alcohol or other substance abuse, evenings or weekends may have been especially difficult or perhaps a mix of maniacally fun and dangerous. Consider how it felt then and how you may be continuing those patterns in some ways now. Are you habitually late in the morning? Do you dread family dinners? Is your substance use feeling out of your control?

As you reflect on particularly triggering times of the day, week, or year, try to find ways to replace those negative patterns with positive ones. If mornings have been chaotic for you, take steps to bring calmness to your morning routine, for example by reading the paper, doing yoga, or walking to work. If your birthdays have been stressful, do something to celebrate that feels good to you. Instead of seeing your family, see a few friends or go out of town. The point is that you no longer have to allow your parents, family, or past to dictate how you organize your life.

 FOOD FIGHTS

For Jade, dinners became stressful when her mother remarried and her narcissistic stepfather took over the cooking. He ridiculed her almost every night about being a picky eater. "I didn't like vegetables or trying new things, and it infuriated him," Jade said. "My parents had never cared, but to him it became a character indictment, like I was a spoiled brat who didn't appreciate what I had or the finer things in life." For a long time, Jade felt ashamed and angry, and as an adult she continued to refuse to eat most vegetables. "I was still carrying anger about it and trying to exert some control," she said. "I understand now that he felt personally insulted when I didn't eat everything on my plate." These days, at nearly 40, she eats vegetables with her 3-year-old twins. "We're making it fun together, and that has been very healing." ‹‹

Let Go of the Need to Be Right

In narcissistic families, being "right" is the golden crown narcissists wear as evidence that they reign supreme. In their mind—to sustain their self-esteem—they must be right and others must be wrong. They have so much at stake in being right that they contort themselves to make it be so, often against all reason. If someone else is shown to be right in a way narcissists can't directly dispute, they may try to position themselves in alliance with the "right" person or take ownership of their "rightness." As the child of a narcissist, you have been taught in a range of ways that you are either wrong or you are right in partnership with the narcissistic parent. In your experience, being wrong or just perceived as wrong opens you up to judgment and possibly ridicule. Naturally, being wrong may feel shameful and dangerous to you. You may have spent a great deal of energy in your life trying to be right without understanding why.

Confronting this fear and possible compulsion is necessary for your emotional health. The narcissistic personality cannot face being wrong, but you can. Getting facts right is often important, but the need to be right should end there. We're all wrong from time to time about many things, and it need not be an indictment of our fundamental human worth. For narcissists, it is, but for emotionally stable people, being right is not the point. Being kind, being truthful with ourselves and others, and being connected matter so much more. Being loving always trumps rightness. Let yourself be fully human, which means allowing yourself to be wrong.

Allow Yourself Success and Failure

Success and failure are major issues for narcissists, who must see themselves as exceptional in some way to avoid feeling like abject failures. Children in narcissistic homes struggle with complicated messages about achievement that are tied to their parents' distorted beliefs. Typically, narcissistic parents have rigid and/or superficial ideas of success and failure that they expect their children to conform to. Such ideas are also commonly tied to the roles such children play in the family. Children may feel pressure to excel at just about everything, to excel in specific ways but not others, to do well enough but not too well, or to not succeed at all. Children from families that identify as high achieving usually feel they have to excel or excel in a particular way to be accepted. The hero or golden child typically feels pressure to achieve in areas valued by the parents but also may receive the message not to outshine them. The lost child may be expected to remain in the shadow of the favored child, while the mascot may be given license to pursue his or her own "cute" or "wacky" interests. Often the scapegoated child is expected to fail where the golden child excels, while the scapegoat's areas of achievement are dismissed or devalued. When children do not conform to parents' expectations, they may be ignored or punished, or find themselves cast in a different family role.

Adult children of narcissists (ACoNs) often find themselves pursuing goals or careers that their parents pushed for them in one way or another only to realize, sometimes late in life, that those things are not what they want. No matter who you are in the family system, you are likely to be confused about your abilities and ambivalent about success. You probably hold yourself to unrealistically high or low standards. A fear of failure can make you highly competitive and perfectionist or lead you to give up or not even try. Similarly, a fear of success can compel you to hold back or sabotage yourself. Whether you succeed or fail, you may feel numb or like an impostor because you are alienated from yourself and your own interests and values. "Failing" feels humiliating, but "succeeding" feels empty, fraudulent, or dangerous.

As an ACoN, you need a paradigm shift in how you understand so-called success and failure. Both of these are subjective and fleeting states that are interconnected and offer helpful lessons in our lives. What we call failure teaches us what does not work and enables us to hone our understanding and skill. There is no success without it. And success is merely a state of achievement that reflects our growth and mastery, not our intrinsic worth. Like failure, success is part of the process of growing, not the point of it. When success is the goal, growth stops. As long as we are succeeding *and* failing, we continue to change and grow.

As an ACoN, it is also important for you to recognize that there are probably areas of yourself that are overdeveloped and areas that are underdeveloped. You may be, for example, highly proficient professionally but struggle in your personal life. Maybe you are gifted at helping others but neglect your own needs. Perhaps you excel at logical and linear tasks but are disconnected from emotional, artistic, or spiritual dimensions of yourself.

Try not to judge yourself for the imbalances in your life. As we know, the narcissistic family is characterized by distortions and extremism. Take the opportunity now to explore aspects of yourself that may have been discouraged or suppressed. As you work on healing, give yourself permission to redefine your values and what success means to you now.

Be Aware of Your Attractions with Narcissists

Adult children of narcissists are vulnerable to being drawn into situations or relationships with narcissists beyond their family of origin, including partners, friends, teachers, and bosses. As we have discussed previously, coming from such a family predisposes you to narcissistic relational dynamics. So, pay attention to the patterns and signs. Try not to jump into jobs and relationships. When someone triggers emotions in you, positive or negative, s/he may be interacting with you as your family did/does. If you're exhilarated, it could be because you're feeling the kind of reinforcement that passed for love in your family. If you're feeling exposed or rattled, it may be an area of hurt or shame stemming from your family. Practice stepping back and examining how you feel and why. This is an opportunity to gain insight and change your patterns. If something feels off, it probably is. If you get tripped up in an unhealthy drama, forgive yourself and move on. In time, you will develop a fine-tuned "nardar." There are a lot of people out there with stable personalities, so go find them!

DEAL BREAKER

Brad grew up in a narcissistic family, so it wasn't surprising that his childhood best friend was narcissistic. "Sandy had been abandoned by his father, and his mother and brother were narcopaths," Brad said. "Sandy was leaps and bounds better than his family and over the years he tried to work on himself, so I overlooked a lot that was wrong with the friendship." Brad forgave Sandy for crashing his car and bailing on him when Brad's parents divorced, but excusing Sandy got harder as they got older. Then, Brad's son was diagnosed with cancer. "I hesitated to tell Sandy because I figured he wouldn't respond well and that was a deal breaker for me. When finally I told him about the cancer, he made a lame attempt at sympathy and quickly changed the subject back to himself. This was the guy who wanted to be my child's godparent," Brad recalled. "After over 20 years of friendship, I just hung up the phone and haven't talked to him since." «

Honor Your Feelings about Your Narcissistic Parent

Most of us love our parents no matter what, and we cling to our need for love and validation from them. Your narcissistic parent cannot love you unconditionally the way we all deserve to be loved within our families, and for that matter is only capable of intermittent affection or concern, if that. Yet you may still love that parent. Your grief and anger may be mixed with sympathy for your parent. It is also possible that you are numb to your parent or too used up to feel love anymore.

Whatever you feel, try not to judge yourself for it. Honor your feelings and let them be your guide in how you choose to interact with your family. Go no contact if that feels like the safest choice. Or operate with firm boundaries and lowered expectations. Narcissistic parents, unless they are sadistic, are usually capable of affection for their children when it doesn't conflict with their own needs. Your parent may be able to give at times and in ways that you find nurturing or helpful. This is most likely to happen when the narcissistic parent is not threatened and derives self-esteem from playing a positive role in your life. With a healthy dose of skepticism, take the good when it comes, as limited and fleeting as it may be.

Write a Letter to Your Narcissistic Parent

Writing is a powerful tool for processing emotions. It can help us identify our feelings and get to the root of where they come from. Children from narcissistic families have a profound need to express their emotions because they have in effect been silenced by their parents. In the narcissistic family, free expression is a privilege reserved for the narcissist(s), while children's expression is equivalent to sacrilege. As you work to understand your feelings and give validity and voice to them, writing can be a great ally. Try to set aside your inner critic and editor. Your writing is for you and need not be "good" or "correct."

Try writing an honest letter to your parent. Chances are, you have never been honest with her/him. This is your opportunity to say what you have not been allowed to say. Give yourself permission. Work on it as long as you like. You need not send the letter; the point is to give it free expression. If you are thinking of sending it, put it away for a week first. After that time has passed, return to the letter and decide whether you actually want to send it and deal with the fallout. Remember that your letter is unlikely to change anything in your family and could inflame things. The important part is writing it. If you have someone in your life you trust with your feelings about your family, you might find it helpful to share it with that person.

If this process helps you, you may want to write more letters to that parent or perhaps to other family members. Make sure to give yourself time before you decide whether to send them. The heat of the moment is not the time to press send or slip an envelope into the mail.

 WRITING CATHARSIS

Magda's therapist had been encouraging her to acknowledge her mother's narcissism. Her mother was alive and well, but Magda found herself thinking about what she would say after her death in a eulogy. When she sat down to write it, she was shocked at how negative her feelings were, but she allowed herself to fully vent and not feel guilty. "After I wrote that negative eulogy, I felt so much better. I knew I would never deliver it, but it really helped me admit what I had been afraid to face," she said. ‹‹

Keep a Journal

Writing can be a highly therapeutic way to gain self-awareness. Talk to any committed writer and s/he will tell you that meaningful writing is always a process of discovery. Take time regularly to record your thoughts and feelings in a journal. It need not be great literature or profoundly insightful. Just write whatever comes to mind as a way to stay connected with yourself and process your experience as you work on healing. Try using actual paper instead of doing it on a computer or other device. The physical act of putting pen to page and writing out thoughts in longhand is a visceral experience that helps us access our emotions. If you want, treat yourself to a beautiful journal and your favorite kind of pen.

Reclaim Your Laughter

We all need to laugh. It literally lifts up our face, releases tension, and elevates our mood. When we have a hearty laugh, we feel connected to life's larger meanings, pleasures, ironies, and truths. Laughter is often a communal experience and one of the most satisfying and bonding things we can share with others.

Yet as someone targeted by a narcissist, you may have experienced laughing as something hurtful, perhaps even dangerous. Narcissists often use laughter as a weapon to control and humiliate. It may be presented as joking or teasing when it is intended manipulatively or punishingly. When we don't laugh along, we are called too sensitive, too serious, humorless. We are punished through the laughter and punished again for not laughing along. When laughter is actually mockery, it is not funny. It is cruelty cloaked as fun. When we are routinely targeted through mocking and demeaning laughter, we come to distrust laughing itself, and in doing so become disconnected from a sustaining part of our humanity.

Laughing is your right and privilege. Taking back your laughter is a vital part of overcoming the narcissist's power over you and reclaiming it for yourself. With people who respect and care about you, you can trust that the laughter is not loaded and pointed at you. You laugh together, not alone. If laughter has been used against you, laughing at yourself may feel too vulnerable. You may have been conditioned to resist it and protect yourself from it. But humor and laughter that you own give you strength. The ability to have a sense of humor about yourself means that you are not afraid or ashamed, as the narcissist is. You don't have to see yourself as perfect, as the narcissist must see her-/himself. You can laugh at yourself freely, generously, and affectionately.

Welcome in the Good about Your Family

Even narcissistic parents and families, with their dysfunction and checkered history, usually have positive elements. There may be family traditions, memories, and experiences you share that you hold dear. You may feel close to some of your family members despite or perhaps because of the tumult you grew up with. Your narcissistic parent may be helpful, funny, smart, talented, or otherwise good to be around at times. In fact, you may be like your narcissistic parent in ways that you value. As you work on understanding and healing from the damage, don't forget to acknowledge the good things about your parents and family. It may take time to sort them out from the painful things, but there will be pieces to hold onto. After all, you wouldn't be you without them.

TRUST YOUR INSTINCTS

Growing up in a narcissistic family is a lonely ordeal. Even if there are siblings, even if there is activity, noise, and drama, you are piercingly alone. You
are alone with your feelings, alone with your needs, alone with your newly
forming body and mind in the ebb and flow of life across the seas of experience with no guide to shore. You have parents, but they are out of reach, cut
off emotionally. You wave and call to them, perform for them, serve them,
perhaps cry and yell for their help, but they don't respond. They look toward
you, talk at you, make demands of you, but *they don't see you.*

You blame yourself for how your parents are. You try to fix yourself, try
to be better, reform, improve, measure up. You begin to compartmentalize
yourself, putting away parts that don't seem acceptable and polishing and
presenting others that might work. You stretch and twist yourself trying to
be the right version of you that will finally get seen, get empathy, get love.

You try for years and then decades to do anything and everything to get
them to see you. Sometimes you feel you've had glimpses, micro moments
of connection that passed as quickly as they came and left you wondering
if they happened at all. You think the problem is you, but it has nothing to
do with you. It never was about you and never will be. You have parents, but
emotionally you are an orphan.

As an adult now, you can set aside denial and self-blame, things the child
does to survive. You can live without parents who see you. It is sad. It is not
an exaggeration to call it a tragedy. It is your family's tragedy, and there is
reason to grieve. Grieving is in fact necessary, as we have discussed. But
you can move on from the tragedy and leave it behind. That is why you are
reading this book—to get help with moving on.

As we know, to move on from complex trauma we must first recognize it
as trauma. Most of us struggle for years believing it is not trauma. But over
time it follows us like a shadow, and the presence of the shadow becomes
darker and heavier. Perhaps we do things to make ourselves forget about the
shadow—compulsive and addictive things, self-defeating things, desperate
things. We run from the shadow, deny its existence, perhaps even recklessly
challenge it to the death, but it is there no matter what we do because it is a
part of us. It is with us when we sleep and when we work. It gets in the way
when we try to play and love.

We know in our gut what we need to do, but we learned long ago to ignore and distrust our instincts. Our parents taught us in countless ways to disown our instincts—the powerful and self-preserving things we feel and know about ourselves, others, and the world around us. What we feel and what we know threaten our insecure and disordered parents. Our integrity and wholeness threaten them, and there is nothing we can do about that. We may not realize it, but our instincts are still there ready to help us. Our integrity is still there, waiting for our full attention. The parts of us that have been disintegrated—pulled apart, distorted, disparaged, and dismissed—are still there waiting to be gathered together and made whole again. We can be whole if we invite them back into our inner conversation and give them the respect they always deserved. We can find our way now as adults if we become alert to our instincts and trust them to guide us where we need to go.

PROCESS YOUR FORESHORTENED SENSE OF THE FUTURE

People who experience trauma often internalize feelings of insecurity and hopelessness about life and their own survival. Children from narcissistic families, particularly ones who are routinely devalued, may carry the sense that their life is precarious and their future is somehow unimaginable, impossible, or doomed. The feeling may be a vague sense that you will die young or not experience a normal lifetime that most people more or less take for granted, or it may be a feeling of impending death. Growing up, you may have had difficulty seeing yourself as an adult and reaching normal milestones such as having a home, committed relationship, job/career, or family. Without even consciously realizing it, you may have believed you were unworthy of or somehow incapable of those things. As an adult, you may carry the persistent belief that your life will be cut short and things you hope for, if you dare to hope, are not possible for you. When other people talk of their future, you may feel a sense of dissociation from your own and marvel at those who have confidence in having full, stable lives.

Your foreshortened sense of your own future is a symptom of CPTSD that comes from direct or implied messages in your family, such as the following:

- Your life is unimportant or worthless.
- There is little or no support for you in the world.

- You can't function on your own.
- You are incapable of having a normal/healthy/good life.
- You can't do what most people can do.
- You'll never be able to hold down a job.
- No one will ever want/love you.
- You don't deserve good things.
- It is wrong/selfish/foolish/dangerous to have goals for yourself.
- You are part of an underclass of the undeserving.
- You aren't smart/attractive/lovable enough to expect happiness or success.
- You are destined to screw up your life.
- Your family will undermine or destroy anything good in your life.
- Everyone in your family is a mess and you are too.
- You can never overcome your past.

Messages like these are devastating to a young person starting out in life. If you are different in some way from your family culture or from societal norms, you are more likely to have received such messages. Narcissistic families are prone to hierarchical, rigid, and intolerant social attitudes, including sexism, queerphobia, ableism, classism, and racism. Even families who espouse open or liberal views often have undercurrents of bigotry. Girls may receive the message that they are expendable. Kids with darker skin may be treated as second rate. LGBTQ teenagers may be kicked out and end up homeless.[3]

In adulthood, illness and financial woes, which often go together and are more common in people with CPTSD, may amplify a foreshortened-future mentality. The instability that frequently comes with physical problems and money worries tends to breed more of the same and creates vicious cycles of disability, unemployment, debt, hopelessness, isolation, and the list goes on.

Doubting your future is a deeply painful and demoralizing state of mind and one that you may have lived with to some extent for years without understanding that it is a result of trauma. You may think you're a pessimist for harboring such feelings or believe that you can't expect better. But a distorted and fatalistic view of your future is not something you have to settle for. It is important for your well-being and for the people who care about you, especially your kids if you have any, that you address this belief system and take steps to move beyond it. What you've experienced is a fundamental loss of faith and feeling of disconnection. Here are some ways to build confidence in your life now and in your future:

- Create a timeline of your major life accomplishments so far. (See the next section on how to do this.)
- Make a photo album or scrapbook of important events/highlights in your life.
- Write down goals you have for the future, including professional and personal goals.
- Make short- and long-term social or travel plans. Challenge yourself to make plans for one week from now, one year from now, and five years from now.
- Read inspirational quotes and stories about people who overcome hardship.
- Join a faith-based organization.
- Challenge yourself to do something you've wanted to do, such as planting a garden, building a deck on your house, taking up drawing, learning another language, or running a marathon.
- Reach out to friends and share your steps with them.

Make an Accomplishments Timeline

Make a timeline of your important accomplishments. Think deeply. Chances are you have more of them than you realize or expected when you were younger. Maybe you earned a degree, learned to play an instrument, overcame a phobia, got a promotion, started a business, kicked cancer, quit drinking, found a loving partner or left an unloving one, or created a family. Remind yourself where you were as a young person and where you've come. How have your achievements exceeded what your parents expected for you? How have they exceeded what you expected for yourself? Right now, as someone actively working on educating yourself and healing, you are taking huge steps that were not possible for you before but are now. Include in your story ways you've worked on healing. Carry this list with you as a reminder of what you are capable of. Read it when you're feeling fearful or hopeless about the future. Over time, make sure to add new accomplishments to your list.

TAKE A SELF-INVENTORY

Coming from a narcissistic family, you have been assaulted in countless ways by your parents' excessive neediness, callous exploitation, and both random and calculated cruelty. You know the giddy high of their idealized attention and the debilitating low of their devaluing and abandoning treatment. Making matters more complicated, you face another difficult reality that extends beyond the pain of dealing directly with their disorder: your own inner narcissist.

Pause. Breathe.

The thought of being like the person who has harmed you to your core can seem like the equivalent of demonic possession. That you might be even somewhat narcissistic like your narcissistic parents feels horrifying, especially if you have played an empathetic or caregiving role in your family and/or if you have been persistently scapegoated. And yet it is nearly inevitable that you will have picked up some of their disordered patterns of thinking, feeling, and behaving. Whether you emulated your parents or not, rebelled against them or not, their modeling influenced you—how you see yourself and how you relate to others. Your ability to break away and heal from the trauma you are carrying depends on your willingness to look at yourself *honestly* and *with compassion*.

Let's back up for a moment. Acknowledging that you took on narcissistic qualities from your parents does not make you responsible for the disordered parenting you received, nor does it mean you are a narcissist. Even if you do suffer from some degree of narcissism, the fact that you are working on understanding yourself with the goal of getting better means *you do not have NPD and you are not stuck*. Remember that narcissism is on a continuum, with diagnosable NPD at one more extreme end. People can change, grow, adapt, learn, and unlearn and do so in endless ways all the time. Cynical statements that people can't change or never change are just that—cynical. A key difference between the narcissist and you, the person working on recovery, is that you are looking at yourself and your life with the goal of being healthier. As we know, narcissists do not do this because they believe they are already perfect. From their perspective, any problems that arise are because of something or someone else. They suffer from a terrible weakness: a rejection of their own humanity.

As the narcissist's child wanting to heal and improve your relationships, you have the strength and will to look at yourself. Take an inventory of your self-defeating narcissistic and codependent patterns. Denying or ignoring them only perpetuates them and is what your parents do. (Read more about codependency in Chapter 13.)

Your Inner Critic/Perfectionist

Ask yourself these questions:
1. Do you dwell on your mistakes and faults?
2. Do you call yourself names?
3. Do you berate yourself?
4. Is it hard to forgive yourself?
5. Do you focus on things you wish you could change about yourself?
6. Do you feel nothing you do is good enough?
7. When you succeed do you immediately raise the bar?
8. Do you have a hard time taking a compliment?
9. Do you focus on the perfect rather than the good enough?
10. Do you strive for ideals that feel out of reach?

If many or most of your answers to these questions are yes, you have a harsh inner critic and perfectionist tendencies. You probably struggle with underlying feelings that you need to prove something and/or earn love or acceptance rather than receive it unconditionally. These are very common issues for people from narcissistic families. You have internalized your narcissistic parents' hypercriticism of you and others, feeling that nothing you do is good enough because you carry the underlying fear that you are unworthy. In the logic of your family, to not be worthless, you must be perfect—and you are always striving for that unattainable state just to avoid utter personal failure.

Remember that perfectionism isn't the same thing as wanting to do things well. Perfectionism holds us to *impossible standards*. As long as your inner conversation is hypercritical, unfair, and rejecting, nothing you do will be good enough to satisfy yourself. This also affects your relationships. Having an overbearing inner critic often also means you are overcritical of people close to you, or possibly undercritical and too ready to excuse others. Even this self-assessment may make you feel mad at yourself (or me!). That is your parents talking. Try to turn that around into something positive: insight into you that you can use to be kinder, fairer, and happier with yourself. It is your job to be your own best friend.

Your Inner People-Pleaser

Ask yourself these questions:
1. Do you focus on pleasing others more than yourself?
2. Do you look for ways to help people so they will like or need you?
3. Do you have difficulty knowing or saying what you want?
4. Do you see yourself as a caretaker or rescuer?
5. Do you feel uncomfortable or guilty saying no?
6. Do you feel you have to give more than you get in your relationships?
7. When you help people, do you often feel unappreciated or unacknowledged?
8. Do you do things you don't really want to do out of a sense of obligation?
9. Do you worry about other people's enjoyment or happiness?
10. Do you anxiously review social events in your mind for things you did wrong?

If many or most of the answers to these questions are yes, you probably played a hero and/or caregiver role in your family. You place more importance on others' feelings than your own and may be out of touch with what you need or want, feel that it doesn't matter, or expect it won't matter to others. Your sense of identity and self-worth are strongly tied to feeling needed and helping others, but you also struggle with feeling unappreciated for your efforts. Perhaps you've come to expect disappointment but are hurt and resentful about it nonetheless. Setting boundaries such as saying no is difficult for you because you have the underlying belief that if you do you will have no value to others and will therefore end up rejected and alone. Fundamentally, you feel you have to give more and do more to get anything in return. Being the rescuer or fixer can be rewarding, but it is a heavy burden that also leaves you drained because you feel you always have to work for approval and love. These are codependent patterns that are very difficult to avoid for children of narcissists.

The bottom line is that your parents used you to meet their own needs and most likely ignored, rejected, or punished you when you expressed yours. You were taught that your feelings didn't matter and your worth was only what you could do for your parents. You may be extremely capable and adept at helping others, and this has come to define you and your relationships. When you try to assert boundaries, you feel guilty and worried you will lose people. You crave more balance with others, but don't know what that looks like and fear you aren't worthy of it. Try not to act based on feelings of guilt and obligation. Working on your self-awareness and self-esteem apart from doing things for others will help you find more balance. Relying on others and allowing them to help you are ways to build confidence in yourself and establish more genuine intimacy in your relationships.

Your Inner Denier/Dissociator

Ask yourself these questions:
1. Do you avoid talking about your feelings or problems?
2. Are you frequently angry or upset without knowing why?
3. Do your emotions sneak up and surprise you?
4. Do you tend to feel overwhelmed by the emotions of those around you?
5. Do you have trouble identifying what you like or want?
6. Do you feel panicked or annoyed when people talk about their feelings?
7. Do you use drugs or other compulsive behaviors to escape?
8. Does expressing your feelings make you feel uncomfortably vulnerable or weak?
9. Do you dislike people asking you what you feel?
10. Do you push people away when you need help?

If many or most of the answers to these questions are yes, you struggle with self-awareness and tend to deny and disengage from your feelings. Emotions probably feel out of reach, foolish, scary, or even dangerous. Perhaps you see your feelings as having exposed or betrayed you. You may find it easier to express yourself physically or intellectually than emotionally, and it may be frustrating or difficult to talk with others about their emotions.

Your discomfort with feelings has probably made intimacy uneven or troublesome. You may want to get closer to certain people in your life, but don't know how or fear being judged, misunderstood, or rejected. These are natural responses to the emotionally annihilating experience of having narcissistic parents. Your emotional self has been on trial, convicted, and imprisoned. In the narcissistic home, no one but the narcissist is allowed emotional free rein, and shaming children about their feelings is often done with relentless and laserlike precision.

While shutting down our emotional dimension may shield us from attack, it does not ultimately protect us. It insulates us from positive emotions and the profound rewards of intimacy. Boys and men in particular often experience shame about their feelings and resort to emotional disconnectedness. In some ways, girls and women are given more "permission" to express emotion, but they, too, face strong cultural bias against it and messages that emotionality is a dark, irrational, "female" and therefore lesser aspect of our humanness. In reality, our emotions are inseparable from our "thoughts" and guide us in everything we do, even—and especially—when we avoid or devalue them. Regardless of gender, our natural emotional integration is our most powerful state of being and therefore the number one target of the narcissist. As long as we sentence our feelings to a prison cell, we continue to give our narcissistic parents power over us. When we befriend the emotional self and reintegrate it in our life, healing follows.

Your Inner Defendant

Ask yourself these questions:

1. Do you feel frightened, angry, or ashamed when you make mistakes?
2. Do you feel attacked by any form of criticism?
3. Do you constantly cover your bases to avoid appearances of vulnerability or weakness?
4. Do you avoid taking responsibility because you don't want to be blamed for bad outcomes?
5. Do you exaggerate and overexplain because the facts don't seem persuasive enough?
6. In social situations do you feel uncomfortable or panicked when the focus is on you?

7. Do you feel painfully exposed when you are in a position of public performance?

8. Do you dread and/or avoid situations in which you are evaluated or critiqued?

9. Do you decline opportunities and experiences to avoid exposure and potential embarrassment?

10. Does the thought of appearing foolish feel humiliating to you?

If many or most of the answers to these questions are yes, you feel intensely vulnerable to personal injury and extremely guarded as a result. Mistakes feel shameful, and being seen carries the unbearable risk of humiliation and rejection. Most likely you were heavily judged and blamed in your family, perhaps as the primary scapegoat, and this conditioned you to fear and avoid any form of exposure or vulnerability. You may be talented and ambitious, but your compulsion to protect yourself from potential attack is so strong that you withdraw from opportunities and social connections that could benefit you. Your defensiveness can lead you to misinterpret and push away people who care about you. Your shame about your fears probably escalates your feelings of anxiety, and you may suffer from phobias, such as fear of public speaking. You may find it difficult to laugh at yourself or feel at ease, and criticism or even questioning can feel like an indictment of your fundamental human worth.

Your defensiveness is a direct reflection of the devaluing you endured and perhaps still endure in your family. You may have been attacked your entire life, often for things you had no part in. One way or another you were forced to answer for problems, and there was little to nothing you could do about it. On top of that, you were probably accused of being too sensitive. Defending yourself feels like a way of life that you can't escape, but your efforts to avoid blame make you feel isolated and more ashamed. Even now as an adult, you may feel panic or guilt about things you didn't do.

Healing begins with seeing your experience of being scapegoated for what it really was—cruel, unjust, and not really about you at all. This is much easier said than done, but as long as you continue to doubt and blame the child you were as your family did, you will never be free of the feeling that you are somehow *innately guilty* without motive, evidence, or trial.

When you stop blaming that innocent kid, you will find you can release your fear, end your vigil, and open yourself up to possibilities of who you want to become.

Your Inner Control Freak

Ask yourself these questions:

1. Do you try to anticipate how others will react before you say or do things?
2. Do you try to predict and control possible outcomes?
3. Do you try to make things "perfect"?
4. Do you prefer to have specific plans than be spontaneous?
5. Do you often feel there is a best way to do things?
6. Do you feel panic or frustration when things don't go as planned?
7. Do you try to convince people of your point of view?
8. Do you feel frustrated or angry when people don't agree with you?
9. Do you often feel you are the only person who can get things right?
10. Do you feel responsible when things don't go well?

If many or most of the answers to these questions are yes, you have a strong desire for control and a sense of overresponsibility. You distrust other people's ability to handle potential problems and fear what might happen if you don't manage decisions. You may be quite good at taking the lead and thinking things through, and people in your life may look to you for help in those ways. However, underneath the insistence on control is fear of the disaster that might happen without it.

As we know, the narcissistic family is characterized by emotional chaos. Children in such homes suffer a defining lack of control that is frightening and painful. They become hypervigilant in response to imminent danger. If they can predict bad things before they happen, they may be able to avoid harm or prevent harm to family members. It is natural for such children to look for ways to control their circumstances and to believe they have more control than they do. Trying to manage things can be reassuring in itself because it sustains the possibility of making things better. Anticipating outcomes and avoiding negative consequences can be effective, but when it becomes a compulsion it is burdensome and can distract us from looking at other issues we need to face. Constantly working to control what might happen, we feel responsible for averting danger and responsible when we can't avert it—burdens much too large for any child or adult. We are still driven by fear and the fantasy that we can outsmart natural disaster, and we fall into the trap of taking the blame for things beyond our control.

We need instead to acknowledge the ways in which we were not in control in childhood and the pain and terror of that helplessness. This releases us from responsibility for how we were hurt and allows us to accept our vulnerability then and now. We learn that we can lower our heightened state of vigilance without courting catastrophe. We become more realistic about what we can control in adulthood and open to intimacy with others through shared responsibility.

Be Kind with Yourself

As you conduct your personal inventory, perhaps the most important thing you can do is *be kind with yourself.* Instead of treating these as laundry lists of your flaws or problems, recognize them as ways you adapted to dysfunctional circumstances. Inoculating ourselves with perfectionism is a form of survival. Denying pain and vulnerability is a form of survival. Externalizing our needs by serving others is a form of survival. Avoiding and defending ourselves from attack is a form of survival. Micromanaging our environment is a form of survival. Just as your parents did, you took on certain narcissistic and codependent responses to cope with narcissistic and codependent messages. Sadly, that is how the cycle works. But the cycle ends when you become aware and actively work to change your habits, patterns, and relationships. That is the step your narcissistic parent may not have taken, for whatever reason, and it is the road you're walking on right now.

EMBRACE YOUR VULNERABILITY

For most of us, at times vulnerability can feel uncomfortable, even unsafe. Showing our strength and minimizing our weakness is a natural survival defense that can help us stay alive and meet our needs. But admitting our vulnerability to ourselves and showing it to others are just as important for survival. Being willing to acknowledge our needs and reach out are necessary parts of learning, making friends, having new experiences, and developing intimacy.

Those of us from narcissistic homes experience great turmoil about vulnerability. Our parents have exploited and attacked our vulnerability and modeled denial and hatred of theirs. And perhaps the partners we chose did the same things. It has not been safe for us to express our needs, but as we work on recovery we recognize the importance of doing so and want to be able to without fear or conflict. We have learned the hard way that there is no love without being vulnerable.

As you forge self-awareness, self-acceptance, and self-respect, your relationship with vulnerability naturally evolves. You learn to honor your needs and recognize your ability to open up to others as a form of courage. You come out of hiding, lay down the childhood defenses that bind you in adulthood, and embrace your full humanity and the full humanity of those around you. You recognize the vulnerability in yourself and others as a defining feature of being alive and connected, and you embrace it not as weakness but instead as a sustaining source of strength and fulfillment. Emotional literacy advocate and author Brené Brown explains it this way:

> Vulnerability is the birthplace of love, belonging, joy, courage, empathy, and creativity. It is the source of hope, empathy, accountability, and authenticity. If we want greater clarity in our purpose or deeper and more meaningful spiritual lives, vulnerability is the path.[4]

WELCOME BACK YOUR INNER EXILES

The fundamental experience driving narcissism is shame—feelings of shame, self-doubt, defectiveness, and self-hatred. Shame drives the narcissist's hyperdefensiveness, low self-awareness, impaired empathy, and grandiose compensations. The narcissist exiles parts of her/his authentic self in exchange for a persona s/he adopts in an attempt to get what s/he needs from her/his parents. Those parents don't adapt adequately to her/his needs, so s/he must try to adapt to theirs. This adaptation begins very early in life, as a survival mechanism. But what is meant to support survival becomes dysfunctional as s/he grows older. S/he suffers, and s/he becomes abusive, causing others to suffer. As the child of a narcissist, you have internalized at least some of her/his shame, and it is up to you to do what your parent could not do: make peace with it.

How do you make peace with shame? Shame is like a secret. The more we hide it, the more power it has over us. We defend, lie, rationalize, blame, obfuscate, perfect, deny, and otherwise contort ourselves and the truth along with it, all in fear of our shame. Soon the shame itself becomes bigger than the feeling that caused the shame. What, after all, is the source of the shame?

The list of possible shames is endless, but what it all boils down to is feeling unseen and therefore *not worth seeing*, unloved and therefore *unlovable*. When we face and dissect our shame, we find how irrational it is—how unfair to the self it is. We all belong. We all have something to give. We are all worthy of love.

Consider what parts of yourself you have exiled or banished into hiding. Are they things your narcissistic parent disowned about you? Most likely they are things that parent also disowns about her-/himself. Those parts of you, or selves, are still there: the creative self and the affectionate self, the playful self and the curious self, the open self and the innocent self, the ambitious self, the emotional self, and the needy self. Those parts of you that were ignored, preyed upon, villainized, pathologized, or rejected are still there in you and deserve as much respect and love as any others. Invite them back into your full humanity. It wasn't safe for them when you were a child, but it is now. When you release shame, you find that you don't need to control things, be right, compete, hide, or project an image. You don't need a script to live your life. You don't need to justify or prove yourself to others. You trust yourself, and you are open to yourself. You can share, not exploit. You can say yes or no without conflict. You can give and receive without withholding or coercing.

When we release shame, we naturally also release intolerance and hate. We no longer need to judge and abuse others so they will carry our shame for us. We find that compassion for ourselves builds into compassion for others and all life. We feel connected rather than separate and alienated. We feel gratitude rather than disappointment and resentment. We wish our narcissistic parents could join us in feeling compassionate, connected, and grateful. We see the parts of them in ourselves that we like and value, and we carry that forward in our own lives with our loved ones. We can love our parents, even if they can't quite love us.

twenty-two

Moving On: From Harsh to Healing Lessons

A S YOU LEARN TO RECOGNIZE NARCISSISTIC ATTITUDES AND BEHAVIOR IN your life, you will inevitably see it in your workplace, your community, and society at large. Just as it resides in our families and relationships, it also exists in our schools, our churches, our businesses, and our government. It is alive and well in our systems of communication, news, and entertainment, which serve to both reflect our narcissism and generate more of it. The giant wheel of capitalism turns on narcissistic values and beliefs, selling us shame and its solution: personal perfection for a price. Advertisers tell us we need to fix ourselves, and their products provide the answers to the problems we didn't even know we had. Our teeth are not white enough, nose not straight enough, breasts not big enough, sex not sexy enough, waist too thick, hair too thin, skin too wrinkled, butt too loose or too flat or too wide. We need bigger memory, faster food, larger screens or smaller ones, cooler games, more muscle, less fat, hipper friends, newer houses, bolder and better ideas. We are taught that we are incomplete and unworthy as we are, so we tweak and tone our body and our life, but our soul and spirit wither. Our feelings hide. Our true needs remain unmet.

What do we need? We need affection, warmth, love of self, love shared with others, connections with the Earth, connections with animals and plants. We need good food, clean water and air, safe space to walk and play and laugh, meaningful work. We need to touch and be touched, to listen and be listened to, to sleep and to dream.

The narcissist's shame, self-hatred, intolerance, polarized thinking, re-activity, arrogance, entitlement, hypocrisy, paranoia, competitiveness, lack of compassion, self-involvement, envy, hierarchical thinking, objectification of others, compulsive projecting, desire for power, and need to be right are forms of despair. Despair batters and hollows out the mother, father, and child. The family suffers, and the world suffers. The narcissistic family becomes the world's stage.

LETTING GO AND MOVING ON

Narcissists' impossible mix of primitive neediness, self-focus, and lack of emotional empathy makes them figurative monsters in the lives of those close to them. They drain and hurt family members while expecting them to serve their needs. Their emotional reactivity and compensatory grandiosity and entitlement make them grotesque. And their capacity for emotional harm, vindictiveness, and perhaps also physical violence can be terrifying and downright dangerous.

But although they behave monstrously, narcissistically disordered people are not monsters. They are deeply wounded children who got older. They never had the emotional grounding to love themselves or others. Like anyone else, they deserve decency and compassion. But they do not deserve access to you or permission to keep hurting you. It is your responsibility to protect yourself from their harm, and to help protect those you love from it.

By now, hopefully you understand much more about what you've been through as a survivor of narcissistic abuse, why it is not your fault, and how to let go and move on. Understanding is always the first necessary step as we move toward change.

Forgiveness: What It Is and Why It Matters

There is much talk of forgiveness, but what is it really? Like love, forgiveness begins and ends in your relationship with yourself. You can't love at all without loving yourself. You can't love your cat or your dog or your best friend or your spouse or your child without love for *you*. Love is accepting ourselves and others as we are. Love is something we decide to do each day. Forgiveness at its core is also about acceptance. It is not an excuse or forgetting. It is not permission. It is not even about the person who has wronged you. Forgiveness is your acceptance of your hurt and your release of that hurt. When you forgive, you say, "This happened and it hurt, and now I am finished with the hurt and I release it. I don't harbor resentment or anger. I don't need to punish. As long as I feel anger or the need to seek revenge, the hurt is still in me, and the person who hurt me still has power over me. I forgive, and I let the hurt go. I forgive, and I take my power back. I forgive, and I heal."

In *The Four Agreements*, Don Miguel Ruiz describes forgiveness this way:

We don't have to suffer any longer. First we need the truth to open the emotional wounds, take the poison out, and heal the wounds completely. How do we do this? We must forgive those we feel have wronged us, not because they deserve to be forgiven, but because we love ourselves so much we don't want to keep paying for the injustice.[1]

We hope the narcissist finds a way to accept, love, forgive, and heal, too. But that is not our responsibility, not our journey, and in the end not something we need in order to be able to move on with our own life.

HEALING TAKEAWAYS

Here are some takeaways to remember as you move forward with healing:
1. Narcissistic abuse is emotionally, psychologically, and physically traumatic.
2. How you were treated by the narcissist in your life is not your fault.
3. Narcissists are incapable of unconditional love.
4. Narcissists don't really "see" other people.
5. You are not responsible for narcissists or their behavior.
6. You are responsible for what you do to help yourself move forward.
7. Narcissists are disconnected from themselves.
8. Narcissists may change for the better, but rarely do.
9. Narcissists cannot be reasoned with.
10. To survive, the child must deny abuse.
11. To grow, the adult must overcome denial.
12. Narcissists do not operate with a normal person's moral code.
13. It's not your job to rescue anyone.

14. You can't convince people of things they aren't ready to hear.
15. Healthy boundaries strengthen relationships.
16. Don't assume that others will understand what you've been through.
17. Seek support but also be careful about who you confide in.
18. Get help from a counselor who understands narcissistic abuse trauma.
19. Empathy begets empathy.
20. The desire for vengeance is understandable, but vengeance does not heal.
21. The best "revenge" truly is a life well lived, with love and respect.
22. Our defenses don't have to define us.
23. Having a narcissistic parent does not make you a narcissist.
24. Children from narcissistic families often become highly caring and empathetic.
25. Forgiveness is for you, not the narcissists.
26. Perfection is a lie.
27. No one deserves to be scapegoated.
28. Being the golden child is not actually "golden."
29. Narcissists put their needs before everyone else's, including their children's.
30. Healthy families put children's needs first.
31. Love starts with yourself.
32. Narcissistic trauma often resonates over time from one generation to the next.
33. You can help halt the intergenerational trauma by ending the cycle in your family of choice.
34. Life is not about winning or being right.
35. Fear was never meant to be a way of life.
36. Shame is useless.
37. Humility comes from wisdom and strength.
38. Healing starts with understanding.
39. Everyone belongs, and everyone has value.
40. People with secure self-esteem support democracy more than people who are narcissistic.
41. Overcoming trauma takes time.
42. Your mind, body, and spirit naturally want to heal.
43. Being victimized does not make you a victim.

44. You don't owe a narcissist anything.
45. You don't owe a narcissist's enabler(s) anything.
46. It is never too late to try to make things better for yourself and your kids.
47. Courage is a decision you make each day.
48. Your best is good enough.
49. Love is a renewable resource.
50. The most important lesson narcissists teach is compassion.

As you move beyond the grip of narcissistic parents, partners, or others in your life, remember that you are not alone, you are not destined to repeat unhealthy patterns, and you are capable of healing, joyful freedom, and a higher purpose.

Glossary

TERMINOLOGY RELATING TO PATHOLOGICAL NARCISSISM, NPD, AND NAR-cissistic abuse has been developed by psychologists over decades of treatment and research as well as by survivors of narcissistic abuse trauma seeking a vocabulary to understand and talk about their bedeviling experience. This list is not meant to be exhaustive but rather an overview of some of the terms used in this book.

ACoNs This acronym stands for "adult children of narcissists." It is commonly used by narcissism survivors and those who work with them.

binary thinking A simplistic view that there are only two opposing possibilities in a situation. Because they lack **whole object relations**, narcissists by definition see people and relationships in binary, black-and-white terms.

closet narcissist The closet narcissist manifests NPD in a quieter, less obviously domineering way, typically because s/he grew up in the shadow of an exhibitionist narcissistic parent and was taught that it was unsafe to compete for the spotlight. The closet narcissist is just as grandiose, controlling, and empathy-impaired as the exhibitionist, but seeks status through association and manipulates passive-aggressively.

Cluster B personality disorders Mental health professionals group personality disorders into three clusters. There are four Cluster B personality disorders, including narcissistic personality disorder, antisocial personality disorder, borderline personality disorder, and histrionic personality disorder. Often an individual with one personality disorder will exhibit traits of one or more other disorders.[1]

codependent A condition characterized by alienation from oneself and one's own needs in service to the needs of a narcissistic (or otherwise dysfunctional) personality. The codependent typically takes a caretaking and enabling role with the narcissist, often experiencing an addiction to feelings of being needed and cycles of abuse.

cognitive dissonance A conflict between differing or opposing beliefs or between what we perceive and what we are told is happening. Children and partners of narcissists often experience cognitive dissonance as a result of the narcissist's **gaslighting** messages.

cognitive distortions The narcissistic personality has distorted thinking patterns that interfere with his/her ability to reason, see nuance, be impartial, and judge fairly. Examples of cognitive distortions are personalizing, false dichotomies, and catastrophizing.

cognitive empathy People with NPD usually have normal cognitive empathy, or the ability to recognize what a person is thinking or feeling, but do not engage in emotional empathy.

covert narcissist See **closet narcissist**.

CPTSD The acronym for "complex post-traumatic stress disorder." As opposed to PTSD, which is an anxiety disorder that results from a single traumatic event, CPTSD is a set of symptoms resulting from repeated trauma over months or years, often as a result of abuse by someone in the role of caregiver or protector of the sufferer. Common in narcissistic abuse trauma victims, particularly children and adult children of narcissists, CPTSD includes a wide range of disabling symptoms, including some or all of the following: hypervigilance; generalized fear, anxiety, and agitation; overreactivity; insomnia; nightmares and/or night terrors; self-isolation; difficulty trusting; dissociation; self-destructive behavior; a foreshortened sense of the future; and intrusive thoughts.

denial A fundamental defense mechanism of the narcissistic personality, denial is the unconscious or conscious assertion that a traumatic or abusive event or circumstance did not happen or does not exist, oftentimes even when presented with evidence to the contrary.

devaluation The flipside of the narcissist's **idealization**, devaluation reflects splitting, or seeing oneself and others as either perfect or worthless. Because of their unrealistic expectations, narcissists nearly always come to devalue those they idealize, or they may swing between idealizing and devaluing.

divide and conquer A common strategy of a narcissist, divide and conquer involves sowing divisions among others to weaken and isolate them so they are easier to control.

dysregulation A defining feature of narcissism and those traumatized by narcissistic abuse, dysregulation is an impaired ability to control or modulate one's emotional, psychological, or physiological response to one's environment.

enabler Usually a codependent partner of the narcissist, the enabler normalizes the narcissist's grandiose persona, extreme sense of entitlement, and mistreatment of others by absorbing abuse, acting as an apologist, and often subscribing to her/his view of things.

engulfment A common feature of narcissistic parenting in which the parent subsumes her/his child's identity within her/his own identity. The golden child typically experiences the most engulfment.

exhibitionist narcissist Compared to the closet narcissist, the exhibitionist is outwardly dominating and competitive, loves the spotlight, and demands adoration.

fauxpology A false or disingenuous apology often used by narcissists to pacify, deflect, induce guilt, and/or antagonize. Examples: "I'm sorry you think I'm such a disappointment as a mother," "I'm sorry you interpreted something so innocent as unfair," "I'm sorry you are so sensitive," "I'm sorry you can't understand how others feel," or "I'm sorry you are so angry."

flying monkeys Like the flying monkeys who served the Wicked Witch of the West in *The Wizard of Oz*, flying monkeys in the narcissistic family are enablers who also perpetrate the narcissist's abuse, often to avoid being targeted themselves and/or to benefit from a certain degree of bestowed privilege. Frequently, flying monkeys are narcissistic themselves.

foreshortened sense of the future A symptom of CPTSD that involves a feeling of impending doom or the vague sense that your life will be cut short and/or not include typical milestones that most people experience, such as having a career and family.

gaslighting A form of psychological manipulation in which someone undermines, often systematically, another person's mental state by leading him/her to question his/her perceptions of reality, gaslighting is common in narcissistic families.

golden child A common child role in the narcissistic family, the golden child is singled out for favoritism, typically at the expense of a disfavored, or scapegoated, child.

gray rock A boundary-setting and conflict-avoidance strategy that can be effective in dealing with narcissists in which you make yourself dull and nonreactive, like a colorless, unmoving, impervious rock.

hero A child role in the narcissistic family, the hero becomes an outstanding achiever and/or highly capable rescuer or problem-solver who props up the parents.

hoovering Narcissists often attempt to hoover (as in vacuum suck) people back within their sphere of control through a variety of methods, from promising to reform, to acting unusually solicitous, to dangling carrots, such as gifts or money.

hypervigilance To cope with the emotionally and possibly physically dangerous environment around the narcissist, family members typically become hypervigilant to threat or attack. Hypervigilance drains the body's natural defense system by constantly overloading it. Narcissists themselves are hypervigilant to anything that might trigger their narcissistic defenses.

idealization A form of unrealistic infatuation the narcissistic personality experiences for someone or something that represents the promise of profound love or greatness, idealization is usually followed by **devaluation** and possible abandonment.

infantilization A form of psychological distortion or manipulation common in narcissistic parents that involves treating their children or adult children as younger than they are to undermine, embarrass, and/or otherwise control them, usually to feel needed or superior.

lost child A common role in the narcissistic family, the lost child becomes essentially invisible—quiet, compliant, and undemanding—to placate and avoid attack.

love bombing Slang for describing the narcissistic personality's typical behavior with a new love interest, love bombing reflects the narcissist's infatuation and lack of boundaries and often includes dramatic expressions of ideal love, intense mirroring, unearned intimacy, premature commitment, wild promises, and unrealistic expectations of perfection. Love bombing may be sincere in the moment, or it may be an attempt to hook someone for manipulative reasons.

Machiavellian Cunningly scheming and unscrupulous, following the philosophy of Niccolò Machiavelli that "the ends justify the means."

malignant narcissist A narcissist who derives the self-esteem s/he lacks internally by ruthlessly dominating and abusing others into submission. Attention, adoration, control, and winning are not enough for the malignant narcissist, who seeks also to overpower and humiliate those around her/him.

mascot A common child role in the narcissistic family, the mascot plays the cute or funny "jester" who distracts and diffuses family tensions, is often excused from responsibility and blame, and is not taken seriously.

mirroring Narcissists reflect back other people's behavior and beliefs as a form of copying or in place of intimacy and empathy. In a romantic context, the narcissist's mirroring is often mistaken for affinity, compatibility, and authentic connection.

narcissistic family A dysfunctional family system that typically revolves around the demands of a narcissistic parent and enabling codependent parent (who also may be narcissistic to varying degrees) rather than needs of the developing children. Sometimes the dominant narcissist in the family is a child/sibling. Narcissistic families are characterized by emotional reactivity, extremist thinking, turbulent relationships, denial, distortions, lies, blame, projection, rage, neglect, and other forms of abuse.

narcissistic injury Invalidating emotional experience in childhood that induces shame; interferes with the healthy development of a stable identity, self-esteem, and empathy; and results in narcissistic defense mechanisms. Narcissistic injury also refers to the narcissist's easily triggered underlying shame.[2]

narcissistic personality disorder (NPD) An adaptive defense mechanism against underlying shame and unstable self-esteem, NPD is characterized by grandiose superiority and entitlement; unrealistic fantasies of greatness and/or ideal love; emotional reactivity; envy; distorted thinking patterns; excessive demands for attention and validation; low self-awareness; lack of empathy; and exploitative or abusive behavior.

narcissistic rage The narcissistic personality is hypersensitive to underlying shame and reacts with fury if his/her compensatory persona of superiority and entitlement is threatened.

narcissistic supply Individuals with NPD depend heavily on externalities, such as attention, praise, worth by association, and/or signifiers of status to support their internally deficient self-esteem and unstable sense of identity.

neglect Common in narcissistic families, neglect is a passive form of abuse in which a caregiver ignores the emotional and/or physical needs of her/his dependent(s).

no contact Ending contact with a narcissist is usually the last defense against his/her abuse. For adult children, shutting down communication with narcissistic parents is typically a last resort to protect themselves and their families.

NPD The acronym for **narcissistic personality disorder**.

object constancy The ability to sustain an awareness of overall positive feelings and past positive experiences with people when you are disappointed or hurt by them in some way, or when they are physically absent. When triggered, the narcissist's continuity of perception collapses into present-moment reactive emotion.

out of sight, out of mind See **object constancy**.

overt narcissist See **exhibitionist narcissist**.

parental alienation and **parental alienation syndrome** A disruption of trust and respect in a child/parent relationship that occurs because of an active destabilizing campaign by the other parent. Particularly in divorce or custody dispute scenarios, a narcissistic parent may lead the child to doubt, judge, withdraw from, and/or reject the targeted parent. The narcissistic parent's alienating influence may consist of criticisms that undermine respect and trust, or it may take extreme form as parental alienation syndrome (PAS), in which the child is brainwashed to the point that s/he becomes a participant in the denigration and rejection of the targeted parent.

parentification A common role reversal in narcissistic families whereby parents inappropriately look to children to take on parental responsibilities, often including meeting the parents' emotional and/or physical needs.

projection A defense mechanism very common in people with NPD that involves attributing one's own feelings, actions, or traits to someone else consciously or unconsciously.

PTSD See **CPTSD**.

sadistic narcissism A form of pathological narcissism that includes deriving pleasure from hurting or humiliating others.

scapegoat A common child role in the narcissistic family, the scapegoat is singled out unfairly for disfavored treatment, such as criticism, blame, neglect, unreasonable chores, and restricted freedoms.

schadenfreude From the German *Schaden*, meaning "damage," and *Freude*, meaning "joy," schadenfreude is a feeling of satisfaction or enjoyment in the misfortune of others. The emotion is linked to sadism and the envious and entitled belief that one deserves more and others deserve less.

smear campaign An organized, intentional form of character assassination to discredit someone, often used by narcissists to punish, justify their abuse, or make themselves look superior.

splitting See **whole object relations**.

trauma A deeply distressing or disturbing experience or set of experiences that results in emotional, psychological, and/or physical symptoms.

trauma bond A bond that can form between an abused person and his/her abuser in which the abused becomes physiologically addicted to the roller coaster of positive and negative reinforcement s/he experiences. A trauma-bonded child of a parent abuser is likely to seek out similar relational dynamics and form codependencies with other abusers unless the cycle is broken.

triangulation A common form of narcissistic manipulation in which a person interferes in relationships or brings a third party into a situation to gain leverage. Through triangulation, the narcissist controls the content and exchange of communication, takes things out of context, spreads distortions and lies, and sets up implied or direct negative comparisons.

whole object relations A developmental milestone, whole object relations allows us to see ourselves and others in a complex, nuanced, fully integrated way as having both positive and negative qualities. Narcissists fail to establish whole object relations and are therefore unable to form a stable, realistic view of themselves and others but instead view people in simplistic extremes as either perfect or worthless, without middle ground.

Resources

Recommended Books

The Body Keeps the Score: Brain, Mind, and Body in the Healing of Trauma by Bessel van der Kolk

Borderline, Narcissistic, and Schizoid Adaptations: The Pursuit of Love, Admiration, and Safety by Elinor Greenberg

Childhood Disrupted: How Your Biography Becomes Your Biology, and How You Can Heal by Donna Jackson Nakazawa

Daring Greatly: How the Courage to Be Vulnerable Transforms the Way We Live, Love, Parent, and Lead by Brené Brown

The Drama of the Gifted Child: The Search for the True Self by Alice Miller

The Emperor's New Clothes by Hans Christian Andersen, illustrated by Virginia Lee Burton

The Four Agreements: A Practical Guide to Personal Freedom (A Toltec Wisdom Book) by Don Miguel Ruiz

The Narcissistic Family: Diagnosis and Treatment by Stephanie Donaldson-Pressman and Robert M. Pressman

Stop Caretaking the Borderline or Narcissist: How to End the Drama and Get on with Life by Margalis Fjelstad

This Naked Mind: Control Alcohol, Find Freedom, Discover Happiness, and Change Your Life by Annie Grace

Trauma and Recovery: The Aftermath of Violence—From Domestic Abuse to Political Terror by Judith Herman

Why Does He Do That? Inside the Minds of Angry and Controlling Men by Lundy Bankroft

Will I Ever Be Free of You? How to Navigate a High-Conflict Divorce from a Narcissist and Heal Your Family by Karyl McBride

Will I Ever Be Good Enough? Healing the Daughters of Narcissistic Mothers by Karyl McBride

Books/Films/TV Shows with Narcissistic Characters

Absolutely Fabulous
American Beauty
Arrested Development
Big Eyes
Big Little Lies
Black Swan
Dead Poets Society
The Devil Wears Prada
Doubt
Everybody Loves Raymond
Game of Thrones
Gilmore Girls
Gone Girl
Gone with the Wind
The Great Gatsby
The Great Santini
House of Cards
James and the Giant Peach
Leaving Neverland
Mad Men
Matilda
Mommie Dearest
Mother, Mother
The Office
Ordinary People
The Picture of Dorian Gray
Postcards from the Edge
Precious
Rachel Getting Married
Shameless
Sharp Objects
Six Feet Under
Sleeping with the Enemy
The Sopranos
Sybil
The Tale
The Talented Mr. Ripley
Terms of Endearment
Wall Street
White Oleander

Sources

Introduction

1. Stinson, Frederick S., Deborah A. Dawson, Risë B. Goldstein, S. Patricia Chou, Boji Huang, Sharon M. Smith, W. June Ruan, Attila J. Pulay, Tulshi D. Saha, Roger P. Pickering, and Bridget F. Grant. "Prevalence, Correlates, Disability, and Comorbidity of DSM-IV Narcissistic Personality Disorder: Results from the Wave 2 National Epidemiologic Survey on Alcohol and Related Conditions." *Journal of Clinical Psychiatry* (July 31, 2008). Accessed April 8, 2019. https://www.psychiatrist.com/jcp/article/Pages/2008/v69n07/v69n0701.aspx.

Chapter 1: Understanding Your Rights

1. United Nations. General Assembly. *Universal Declaration of Human Rights: Adopted the 10th December 1948 in Plenary Session by the General Assembly of the United Nations.* UNESCO, 1948.

2. Marchlewska, Marta, Kevin A. Castellanos, Karol Lewczuk, Mirosław Kofta, and Aleksandra Cichocka. "My Way or the Highway: High Narcissism and Low Self-Esteem Predict Decreased Support for Democracy." *British Journal of Social Psychology* (2018). doi:10.1111/bjso.12290.

3. "Stuck in Denial? How to Move on." Mayo Clinic. April 14, 2017. Accessed April 8, 2019. https://www.mayoclinic.org/healthy-lifestyle/adult-health/in-depth/denial/art-20047926.

4. Adapted from United Nations, General Assembly, *Universal Declaration of Human Rights: Adopted the 10th December 1948 in Plenary Session by the General Assembly of the United Nations,* UNESCO, 1948.

Chapter 2: Identifying the Narcissist in Your Life

1. Greenberg, Elinor. *Borderline, Narcissistic, and Schizoid Adaptations: The Pursuit of Love, Admiration, and Safety.* New York: Greenbrooke Press, 2016.

2. Stines, Sharie. "The Arduous Work of Treating Narcissism: A Therapist's Guide." GoodTherapy.org. January 12, 2017. Accessed July 14, 2019. https://www.goodtherapy.org/blog/arduous-work-of-treating-narcissism-therapists-guide-0112174.

3. Interview with Elinor Greenberg. Telephone interview by author. March 20, 2017.

4. Ibid.

Chapter 3: Traits of Narcissistic Personality Disorder

1. Stinson, Frederick S., Deborah A. Dawson, Risë B. Goldstein, S. Patricia Chou, Boji Huang, Sharon M. Smith, W. June Ruan, Attila J. Pulay, Tulshi D. Saha, Roger P. Pickering, and Bridget F. Grant. "Prevalence, Correlates, Disability, and Comorbidity of DSM-IV Narcissistic Personality Disorder: Results from the Wave 2 National Epidemiologic Survey on Alcohol and Related Conditions." *Journal of Clinical Psychiatry* (July 31, 2008). Accessed April 8, 2019. https://www.psychiatrist.com/jcp/article/Pages/2008/v69n07/v69n0701.aspx.

2. Marchlewska, Marta, Kevin A. Castellanos, Karol Lewczuk, Mirosław Kofta, and Aleksandra Cichocka. "My Way or the Highway: High Narcissism and Low Self-Esteem Predict Decreased Support for Democracy." *British Journal of Social Psychology* (2018). doi:10.1111/bjso.12290.

3. Pappas, Stephanie. "Delving into the Mind of a Dictator." LiveScience. February 11, 2011. Accessed April 08, 2019. https://www.livescience.com/12842-delving-mind-dictator-mubarak.html.

4. *Diagnostic and Statistical Manual of Mental Disorders*, 5th ed. Washington, DC: American Psychiatric Association, 2013.

5. Marchlewska, Marta, Kevin A. Castellanos, Karol Lewczuk, Mirosław Kofta, and Aleksandra Cichocka. "My Way or the Highway: High Narcissism and Low Self-Esteem Predict Decreased Support for Democracy." *British Journal of Social Psychology* (2018). doi:10.1111/bjso.12290.

6. Baskin-Sommers, Arielle, Elizabeth Krusemark, and Elsa Ronningstam. "Empathy in Narcissistic Personality Disorder: From Clinical and Empirical Perspectives." *Personality Disorders: Theory, Research, and Treatment* 5, no. 3 (July 2014): 323–333. doi:10.1037/per0000061.

7. Herman, Judith Lewis. *Trauma & Recovery: The Aftermath of Violence: From Domestic Abuse to Political Terror.* New York: Basic Books, 1997, 117–118.

8. Van der Kolk, Bessel. *The Body Keeps the Score: Brain, Mind, and Body in the Healing of Trauma by Bessel Van Der Kolk, MD | Key Takeaways, Analysis & Review.* San Francisco: IDreamBooks, 2015, 145, 166.

9. Hoermann, Simone, and Corinne E. Zupanick. "Problems with the Diagnostic System for Personality Disorders." Mental Help Problems with the Diagnostic System for Personality Disorders Comments. Accessed April 8, 2019. https://www.mentalhelp.net/articles/problems-with-the-diagnostic-system-for-personality-disorders/.

10. Ibid.

11. Ibid.

12. *Diagnostic and Statistical Manual of Mental Disorders*, 5th ed. Washington, DC: American Psychiatric Association, 2013, Section III, Emerging Measures and Models.

13. *Psychodynamic Diagnostic Manual (PDM)*. Silver Spring, MD: Alliance of Psychoanalytic Organizations, 2006.

14. Dimaggio, Giancarlo. "Narcissistic Personality Disorder: Rethinking What We Know." *Psychiatric Times* 29, no. 7 (July 19, 2012). https://www.psychiatrictimes .com/personality-disorders/narcissistic-personality-disorder-rethinking-what-we-know.

15. Seltzer, Leon F. "This Is What Really Makes Narcissists Tick." *Psychology Today*, July 28, 2015. Accessed April 8, 2019. https://www.psychologytoday.com/us /blog/evolution-the-self/201507/is-what-really-makes-narcissists-tick.

16. Fjelstad, Margalis. *Stop Caretaking the Borderline or Narcissist: How to End the Drama and Get On with Life*. Lanham, MD: Rowman and Littlefield, 2014, 18.

17. Seltzer, Leon F. "6 Signs of Narcissism You May Not Know About." *Psychology Today*, November 7, 2013. Accessed April 8, 2019. https://www.psychology today.com/us/blog/evolution-the-self/201311/6-signs-narcissism-you-may-not-know -about.

18. Ibid.

19. Greenberg, Elinor, October 18, 2018. Answer on the question, "If past behavior is the best indicator of future behavior with the narcissist, does this apply to their new relationships too? Will they be as emotionally abusive in the new relationship?" Quora, accessed April 8, 2019. https://www.quora.com/If-past-behavior-is-the -best-indicator-of-future-behavior-with-the-narcissist-does-this-apply-to-their-new -relationships-too-Will-they-be-as-emotionally-abusive-in-the-new-relationship.

20. Greenberg, Elinor. *Borderline, Narcissistic, and Schizoid Adaptations: The Pursuit of Love, Admiration, and Safety*. New York: Greenbrooke Press, 2016.

21. Whitbourne, Susan Krauss. "Do Narcissists of a Feather Flock Together?" *Psychology Today*, May 17, 2016. Accessed April 8, 2019. https://www.psychology today.com/us/blog/fulfillment-any-age/201605/do-narcissists-feather-flock-together.

22. Gregoire, Carolyn. "This Is the Only Personality Type That Enjoys Being with Narcissists." HuffPost. March 14, 2016. Accessed April 8, 2019. https://www .huffpost.com/entry/dealing-with-a-narcissist_n_56e6b177e4b065e2e3d66456.

23. "Narcissism Is a Driving Hazard, Research Suggests." Association for Psychological Science. February 27, 2018. Accessed April 9, 2019. https://www.psychological science.org/news/motr/narcissism-is-a-driving-hazard-research-suggests.html.

24. Seidman, Gwendolyn. "Are Selfies a Sign of Narcissism and Psychopathy?" *Psychology Today*, January 8, 2015. Accessed April 9, 2019. https://www.psychology today.com/us/blog/close-encounters/201501/are-selfies-sign-narcissism-and -psychopathy.

Chapter 4: Causes of Narcissism and the Narcissist's Impaired Empathy

1. "Narcissistic Personality Disorder." Mayo Clinic. November 18, 2017. Accessed April 9, 2019. https://www.mayoclinic.org/diseases-conditions/narcissistic -personality-disorder/symptoms-causes/syc-20366662.

2. "Causes of Narcissistic Personality Disorder (NPD)." Healthdirect. Accessed April 9, 2019. https://www.healthdirect.gov.au/causes-of-npd.

3. Herman, Judith Lewis. *Trauma & Recovery: The Aftermath of Violence: From Domestic Abuse to Political Terror.* New York: Basic Books, 1997, 52.

4. Greenberg, Elinor. *Borderline, Narcissistic, and Schizoid Adaptations: The Pursuit of Love, Admiration, and Safety.* New York: Greenbrooke Press, 2016, 269.

5. Goleman, Daniel. "Three Kinds of Empathy: Cognitive, Emotional, Compassionate." Daniel Goleman. June 12, 2007. Accessed April 9, 2019. http://www.danielgoleman.info/three-kinds-of-empathy-cognitive-emotional-compassionate/.

6. Baskin-Sommers, Arielle, Elizabeth Krusemark, and Elsa Ronningstam. "Empathy in Narcissistic Personality Disorder: From Clinical and Empirical Perspectives." *Personality Disorders* (February 10, 2014). Accessed April 9, 2019. https://www.ncbi.nlm.nih.gov/pmc/articles/PMC4415495/.

Chapter 5: Closet, Exhibitionist, and Malignant Narcissism

1. Greenberg, Elinor. *Borderline, Narcissistic, and Schizoid Adaptations: The Pursuit of Love, Admiration, and Safety.* New York: Greenbrooke Press, 2016, 246.

2. Greenberg, Elinor, May 22, 2018. Answer on the question, "What is covert narcissism?" Quora, accessed April 9, 2019. https://www.quora.com/What-is-covert-narcissism.

3. Diamond, Stephen A. "Is It Narcissism or Sociopathy?" *Psychology Today.* Accessed April 9, 2017. https://www.psychologytoday.com/us/blog/evil-deeds/201707/is-it-narcissism-or-sociopathy.

4. Freeman, Rhonda. "How to Tell You're Dealing with a Malignant Narcissist." *Psychology Today,* February 22, 2017. Accessed April 9, 2019. https://www.psychologytoday.com/us/blog/neurosagacity/201702/how-tell-youre-dealing-malignant-narcissist.

5. Interview with Elinor Greenberg. Telephone interview by author. March 20, 2017.

6. Ibid.

Chapter 6: Narcissistic Abuse

1. Herman, Judith Lewis. *Trauma & Recovery: The Aftermath of Violence: From Domestic Abuse to Political Terror.* New York: Basic Books, 1997, 75–76.

2. Greenberg, Elinor, October 18, 2018. Answer on the question, "If past behavior is the best indicator of future behavior with the narcissist, does this apply to their new relationships too? Will they be as emotionally abusive in the new relationship?" Quora, accessed April 9, 2019. https://www.quora.com/If-past-behavior-is-the-best-indicator-of-future-behavior-with-the-narcissist-does-this-apply-to-their-new-relationships-too-Will-they-be-as-emotionally-abusive-in-the-new-relationship.

3. Singer, Margaret. "Psychological Coercion." *Psychological Coercion* (2011). Accessed April 9, 2019. https://theneurotypical.com/psychological_coercion.html.

Chapter 7: The Health Fallout of Narcissistic Trauma

1. Van der Kolk, Bessel. *The Body Keeps the Score: Brain, Mind, and Body in the Healing of Trauma by Bessel Van Der Kolk, MD | Key Takeaways, Analysis & Review.* San Francisco: IDreamBooks, 2015, 59, 81.

2. Ibid., 30.

3. Herman, Judith Lewis. *Trauma & Recovery: The Aftermath of Violence: From Domestic Abuse to Political Terror.* New York: Basic Books, 1997, 119.

4. Van der Kolk, B. A. "The Compulsion to Repeat the Trauma. Re-enactment, Revictimization, and Masochism." Psychiatric Clinics of North America. June 1989. Accessed April 10, 2019. https://www.ncbi.nlm.nih.gov/pubmed/2664732.

5. Herman, Judith Lewis. *Trauma & Recovery: The Aftermath of Violence: From Domestic Abuse to Political Terror.* New York: BasicBooks, 1997, 36.

6. Interview with Regina Collins. Telephone interview by author. April 12, 2016.

7. Ibid.

8. Interview with Julie Tenenberg. Telephone interview by author. April 13, 2016.

Chapter 8: Rules and Roles in the Narcissistic Family

1. Moon, Tom. "Dysfunctional Family Roles." Tom Moon MFT. 2017. Accessed April 10, 2019. http://www.tommoon.net/?s=roles.

2. Donaldson-Pressman, Stephanie, and Robert M. Pressman. *The Narcissistic Family: Diagnosis and Treatment.* San Francisco: Jossey-Bass Publishers, 1997, 30.

3. Ibid.

4. *Ordinary People.* Directed by Robert Redford. Performed by Mary Tyler Moore, Timothy Hutton. September 19, 1980. Accessed April 10, 2019.

5. Wegscheider-Cruse, Sharon. *Another Chance: Hope and Health for the Alcoholic Family.* Palo Alto, CA: Science and Behavior Books, 1989.

6. Whitbourne, Susan Krauss. "Can Two Narcissists Ever Really Fall in Love?" *Psychology Today*, September 5, 2017. Accessed April 10, 2019. https://www.psychologytoday.com/us/blog/fulfillment-any-age/201709/can-two-narcissists-ever-really-fall-in-love.

7. Interview with Elinor Greenberg. Telephone interview by author. March 20, 2017.

8. Van der Kolk, Bessel. *The Body Keeps the Score: Brain, Mind, and Body in the Healing of Trauma by Bessel Van Der Kolk, MD | Key Takeaways, Analysis & Review.* San Francisco: IDreamBooks, 2015.

Chapter 9: Patterns in the Narcissistic Family

1. Herman, Judith Lewis. *Trauma & Recovery: The Aftermath of Violence: From Domestic Abuse to Political Terror.* New York: Basic Books, 1997, 75.

2. Szalavitz, Maia. "Why We're Psychologically Hardwired to Blame the Victim." *Guardian,* February 27, 2018. Accessed April 10, 2019. https://www.theguardian.com/us-news/2018/feb/27/victim-blaming-science-behind-psychology-research.

3. Poulsen, Alison. "Positive Projection: 'He Is So Amazingly Intelligent and Articulate!'" Couples Solutions. March 29, 2012. Accessed April 10, 2019. https://www.sowhatireallymeant.com/2011/10/18/positive-projection-"he-is-so-amazingly-intelligent-and-articulate"/.

Chapter 12: Romance, Partnership, and Breakup with a Narcissist

1. Herman, Judith Lewis. *Trauma & Recovery: The Aftermath of Violence: From Domestic Abuse to Political Terror.* New York: Basic Books, 1997, 82.

2. Greenberg, Elinor. *Borderline, Narcissistic, and Schizoid Adaptations: The Pursuit of Love, Admiration, and Safety.* New York: Greenbrooke Press, 2016, 256.

3. Libersat, Frederic, Maayan Kaiser, and Stav Emanuel. "Mind Control: How Parasites Manipulate Cognitive Functions in Their Insect Hosts." Frontiers. April 4, 2018. Accessed April 10, 2019. https://www.frontiersin.org/articles/10.3389/fpsyg.2018.00572/full.

Chapter 13: Codependency and Narcissism

1. Herman, Judith Lewis. *Trauma & Recovery: The Aftermath of Violence: From Domestic Abuse to Political Terror.* New York: Basic Books, 1997, 92.

2. Van der Kolk, B. A. "The Compulsion to Repeat the Trauma. Re-enactment, Revictimization, and Masochism." Psychiatric Clinics of North America. June 1989. Accessed April 10, 2019. https://www.ncbi.nlm.nih.gov/pubmed/2664732.

3. Ibid.

4. "Top Ten Indicators That You Show Signs of Codependency." Recovery Connection. December 13, 2018. Accessed April 10, 2019. https://www.recoveryconnection.com/top-ten-indicators-suffer-codependency/.

5. Herman, Judith Lewis. *Trauma & Recovery: The Aftermath of Violence: From Domestic Abuse to Political Terror.* New York: Basic Books, 1997, 75.

6. Andersen, Hans Christian. *The Emperor's New Clothes.* Folk Tale Classics. New York: HMH Books for Young Readers, 2004.

Chapter 15: Parenting with a Narcissist

1. Stines, Sharie. "Children with Attachment Based Narcissistic 'Parental Alienation Syndrome.'" *Psych Central.* May 12, 2017. Accessed April 10, 2019.

https://pro.psychcentral.com/recovery-expert/2016/06/children-with-narcissistic
-parental-alienation-syndrome/.

Chapter 16: The Under- and Overparented Child

1. Teicher, Martin H., and Gordana D. Vitaliano. "Witnessing Violence toward Siblings: An Understudied but Potent Form of Early Adversity." *PloS One* (December 21, 2011). Accessed April 10, 2019. https://www.ncbi.nlm.nih.gov/pmc/articles /PMC3244412/.

2. "Child Welfare Outcomes 2015." National and State Child Abuse and Neglect Statistics—Child Welfare Information Gateway. Accessed April 10, 2019. https://www.childwelfare.gov/topics/systemwide/statistics/can/can-stats/.

Chapter 17: Understanding and Overcoming Your Family Role

1. *Leaving Neverland.* Directed by Dan Reed. January 25, 2019. Accessed April 10, 2019. https://www.hbo.com/documentaries/leaving-neverland.

Chapter 19: Processing Your Trauma

1. Herman, Judith Lewis. *Trauma & Recovery: The Aftermath of Violence: From Domestic Abuse to Political Terror.* New York: Basic Books, 1997, 114.

2. Goode, Erica. "The World; Stalin to Saddam: So Much for the Madman Theory." *New York Times*, May 4, 2003. Accessed April 10, 2019. https://www .nytimes.com/2003/05/04/weekinreview/the-world-stalin-to-saddam-so-much-for -the-madman-theory.html.

3. "The Real Idi Amin." www.newvision.co.ug. October 12, 2012. Accessed April 10, 2019. https://www.newvision.co.ug/new_vision/news/1307958/real-idi-amin.

4. Stirling, John, and Lisa Amaya-Jackson. "Understanding the Behavioral and Emotional Consequences of Child Abuse." *Pediatrics* (September 1, 2008). Accessed April 10, 2019. https://pediatrics.aappublications.org/content/122/3/667.

5. Ibid.

6. McBride, Karyl. *Will I Ever Be Good Enough?* New York: Simon & Schuster, 2008, 144.

7. Feldman, David B. "Why the Five Stages of Grief Are Wrong." *Psychology Today*, July 7, 2017. Accessed April 10, 2019. https://www.psychologytoday.com /us/blog/supersurvivors/201707/why-the-five-stages-grief-are-wrong.

8. "Why Experts Talk about Symptoms, Not Stages, of Grief." Crossroads Hospice and Palliative Care. August 30, 2017. Accessed April 10, 2019. https:// www.crossroadshospice.com/hospice-palliative-care-blog/2017/august/30/ why-experts-talk-about-symptoms-not-stages-of-grief/.

9. Smith, Claire Bidwell. *Anxiety: The Missing Stage of Grief: A Revolutionary Approach to Understanding and Healing the Impact of Loss.* New York: Da Capo Press, 2018, 20–21.

10. Ibid.

11. Ibid., 76.

12. Ibid., 76–84.

13. Van der Kolk, B. A. "The Compulsion to Repeat the Trauma. Re-enactment, Revictimization, and Masochism." Psychiatric Clinics of North America. June 1989. Accessed April 10, 2019. https://www.ncbi.nlm.nih.gov/pubmed/2664732.

14. Ibid.

15. Interview with Fiona Steele. Telephone interview by author. April 14, 2016.

16. Interview with Regina Collins. Telephone interview by author. April 12, 2016.

17. Interview with Karyl McBride. Telephone interview by author. April 18, 2016

18. Interview with Sharone Weltfreid. Telephone interview by author. July 15, 2019.

Chapter 21: Steps to Recovery

1. Miller, Alice. *The Drama of the Gifted Child*. New York: Basic Books, 1997, 81.

2. Louv, Richard. *Last Child in the Woods: Saving Our Children from Nature-Deficit Disorder*. London: Atlantic Books, 2013.

3. "LGBT Homelessness." National Coalition for the Homeless. Accessed April 10, 2019. https://nationalhomeless.org/issues/lgbt/.

4. Brown, Brené. *Daring Greatly: How the Courage to Be Vulnerable Transforms the Way We Live, Love, Parent, and Lead*. New York: Avery, 2015.

Chapter 22: Moving On: From Harsh to Healing Lessons

1. Ruiz, Miguel. *The Four Agreements: A Practical Guide to Personal Freedom*. Toronto, CNIB, 2006, 114–115.

Glossary

1. Salters-Pedneault, Kristalyn. "Understanding Cluster B Personality Disorders in the DSM-5." Verywell Mind. March 21, 2019. Accessed April 10, 2019. https://www.verywellmind.com/the-cluster-b-personality-disorders-425429.

2. Dimaggio, Giancarlo. "Narcissistic Personality Disorder: Rethinking What We Know." *Psychiatric Times* 29, no. 7 (July 19, 2012). https://www.psychiatrictimes.com /personality-disorders/narcissistic-personality-disorder-rethinking-what-we-know.

Index

name dropping, as narcissistic "quirk," 33
narcissism, as abusive disorder, 55–56
narcissist, as narcissistic family role, 79
The Narcissist Family Files (blog), xix
narcissistic abuse. *See* abuse, narcissistic
narcissistic families. *See* families,
    narcissistic
The Narcissistic Family (Donald-
    Pressman and Pressman), 73–74
narcissistic injury, 28, 272
narcissistic personality disorder (NPD),
    13–69. *See also* traits of narcissistic
    personality disorder
  aging narcissists, 228–230
  causes of narcissism and the narcissist's
    impaired empathy, 38–46
  characteristics, 272
  closet, exhibitionist, and malignant
    narcissism, 47–53
  as Cluster B personality disorder, 15, 22
  defined, 17–18, 272
  diagnosis, 10–12, 18
  health fallout of narcissistic trauma,
    63–69
  impaired empathy, 43–44
  introduction, xxi
  narcissistic abuse, 54–62
  narcissistic supply, 273
  prevalence, xvii, 15
  projection, 273
  as spectrum disorder, 15, 47
  stigma surrounding, 11
  therapy and, 10–11
  why an official diagnosis of NPD is
    unlikely, 10–11
narcissistic supply, 19, 273
The Narcissist You Know (Burgo), 26
nature, in healing strategy, 242
negative projection, 96–97
neglect
  of children of narcissists, 169–172
  defined, 169, 273
  learning not to need, 170–172
  overindulgence as, 175
  types of, 169–170

niceness, when the narcissist is nice,
    220–221
no contact, 227–228, 273
NPD. *See* narcissistic personality
    disorder

object constancy, 24–25, 273
On Death and Dying (Kübler), 208
online narcissists, 34–36
only children, 168
Ordinary People (movie), 77–78
out of sight, out of mind. *See* object
    constancy
overcoming narcissistic abuse, 201–268.
    See also recovery steps; trauma
    processing
  breaking family pattern of narcissism,
    116–118
  introduction, xxii
  leaving your narcissistic partner,
    143–146
  managing the narcissist in your life,
    220–233
  moving on: from harsh to healing
    lessons, 264–268
  overcoming codependency, 136–137
  understanding your anger, 8–9
overgeneralizing, 107
overindulgence, 175–177
overpraising, 177–178
overt narcissist. *See* exhibitionist
    narcissist

parallel parenting with a narcissist ex,
    159–162. *See also* managing the
    narcissist in your life; parenting
    with a narcissist
  document, document, document, 162
  do list, 161
  don't list, 161–162
  forget coparenting and accept parallel
    parenting, 160–161
  your narcissist ex doesn't love your
    kids the way you do, 159–160
parasites, narcissists as, 124, 129–130